Coronary Artery Disease

Genes, Drugs and the Agricultural Connection

Coronary Artery Disease

Genes, Drugs and the Agricultural Connection

Ole Færgeman

2003

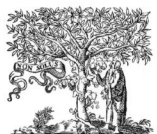

ELSEVIER

ELSEVIER SCIENCE B.V.
Sara Burgerhartstraat 25
P.O. Box 211, 1000 AE Amsterdam, The Netherlands

First edition 2003

Library of Congress Cataloging in Publication Data
A catalog record from the Library of Congress has been applied for.

British Library Cataloguing in Publication Data
Coronary artery disease: genes, drugs and the agricultural connection
    1. Coronary heart disease 2. Coronary heart disease – Etiology 3. Coronary heart
    disease – Treatment
      I. Faergeman, Ole
      616.1'23

ISBN: 0-444-51382-5 (Hardbound)
        0-444-51396-5 (Paperback)

∞ The paper used in this publication meets the requirements of ANSI/NISO Z39.48-1992 (Permanence of Paper).
Printed in The Netherlands.

For Marion Jespersen

Foreword

This book is about coronary heart disease. But that would be to demean its real value. Ole Færgeman has brought together from innumerable sources information which places coronary artery disease in a historical, evolutionary, and scientific context. The book is eminently readable by both the lay public and members of the medical profession.

The life expectancy in most of the high-income countries in the world increased in the last century from about 40 years towards 80 years. That is a quite remarkable achievement and was the consequence partly of the explosion of medical knowledge and partly of changes in social organisation resulting in cleaner water, better housing and access to a reasonable diet. The pattern of disease changed from infection to chronic diseases. Across the world the same pattern is emerging. In the poorer countries infection, malaria, AIDS and tuberculosis remain the main causes of death, whereas in the middle income countries, accounting for 60% of the world's population, there is an explosion in what are called non-communicable diseases. The public might regard those as chronic diseases. The two most important are heart disease and stroke. Both have their origins in disease processes within the walls of arteries and in the many and various abnormalities in the constituents of the blood. Though the simple risk factors linked to heart attacks and strokes are known, namely smoking, hypertension, diabetes and lipid abnormalities, the underlying causes are only just emerging. What is clear is that alterations in the state of society in general are major contributions to these well-known risk factors. For example, urbanisation in India is accompanied by increasing obesity, diabetes and hypertension. Thus, the fundamental causes of disease are modified by political change impacting on the way in which people are housed and live and the food to which they have easy access at reasonable cost. Although there is evidence that some genetic abnormalities contribute to the development of coronary heart disease and in particular there may be genes which have provided advantage to particular peoples in particular parts of the world over past ages and now are harmful by increasing the propensity to heart disease, most of heart disease is preventable and relates to how society is organised and to known risk factors.

Physicians and health workers often fail to appreciate the historical and scientific context of disease. That is because they are critically involved in the day to day management of patients. This book makes the topic exciting and provides extraordinary insight into the importance of history and how science, society and social circumstances interact.

Philip A. Poole-Wilson

Acknowledgments

I wrote most of this little book when the Danish Heart Foundation gave me the means (grant no. 22511) to spend ten months, five before and five after, the turn of the century, at the University of California in San Francisco. I was a visitor in the laboratory of my friend, Henry R. Bourne, and Henry as well as other good friends in the United States, Richard J. Havel, John B. Newell and Ernst J. Schaefer, in particular, provided valuable advice after reading early versions of the manuscript. Later versions were substantially helped by criticism from Axel Bonde, Edith Clausen, Ulrik Gerdes, Thorkild Kjærgaard, Larry S. Liebovitch, Michael F. Oliver, Bent Raungaard, and my son, Thomas Færgeman. I am grateful to them all. They must not be blamed for any mistakes the reader might find, nor should they be held accountable for the points of view that I advance in this book. Discussions that I have had with Charlie Sing and with my closest collaborators over two decades have deeply informed those points of view. In addition to people already mentioned, those collaborators include Lone Andersen, Lars Bolund, Dorte Damgaard, Christian Gerdes, Niels Gregersen, Peter Steen Hansen, Finn Health, Henrik Kjærulff Jensen, Jesper Møller Jensen, Lillian G. Jensen, Ib Christian Klausen, Steen Kølvraa, Mogens Lytken Larsen, Lone Lemming, Jens Uffe Brorholt Petersen and Vibeke Reiche Sørensen.

I am very grateful to Elizabeth Harding for editing the text, and I wish to thank Mia Lejsted for suggesting to me that the Ymer Well by the Danish sculptor, Kai Nielsen, could serve as a cover illustration. The sculpture stands in Faaborg Museum, and I am grateful to Susanne Thestrup Truelsen for access to a good photograph. It conveys the whole idea, but I hope you will read the book for a bit of elaboration.

Aarhus, March, 2003

Ole Færgeman

Contents

Introduction

The Korean War ended in 1953. That year American military pathologists published a report which briefly caused widespread public concern.[1] They had performed autopsies on soldiers killed in action in order to understand combat injuries better, and to ascertain how physicians might improve their treatment of them. The pathologists also happened to look at the blood vessels that had supplied the hearts of the young men with oxygen and nutrients. These are the coronary arteries. It turned out that the coronary arteries of most of the dead soldiers were not at all normal. They had been deformed by atherosclerosis. The disease had almost certainly not caused any symptoms, but had those young soldiers survived the war, most of them would have had symptoms of heart disease later on, and they would have been likely to die of a heart attack.

Since then, many other studies have confirmed that atherosclerosis of the arteries is extremely common many years before symptoms appear. None of the studies had much impact on the way we practice medicine, however, because they had all been performed on dead people. That is changing. New kinds of x-ray machines, echocardiography machines, and magnetic resonance scanners enable physicians to see whether or not a living person has disease of the coronary arteries and how extensive it is. Whereas the pathologist could only record his findings, a physician responsible for living patients must decide what to do about a disease that he has detected.

It is not hard to guess what he will do. He has been trained to treat disease, and it is fairly certain that the person, now a patient, will want to be treated. Since we know that physicians will detect atherosclerosis in many people over the age of 30 years and in almost everyone over the age of 60 years, a very large proportion of the populations of all affluent countries is going to be treated with drugs for coronary artery disease, even if the disease has not yet caused any symptoms. Improved ability to detect coronary artery disease is just one part of the story that is emerging at the beginning of the 21st century. The European Society of Cardiology has called the disease "Today's Black Death", and in the summer of 2002 it presented a "Heart Plan for Europe" to the Council of the European Union. The plan is an ambitious one. For example, it calls for reduction of blood cholesterol in individuals to 5 mmol/l by 2007.[2] In many countries, however, far more than half of the population have cholesterol levels above this level. If drug treatment of most of the population is to be avoided, we must think harder about other remedies.

"Today's Black Death" is also becoming more common across the planet. The World Health Organization expects that, by 2020, coronary artery disease will head the list of diseases burdening the health systems of the world. We know a lot about the causes of this disease. We have also learned a lot about how to treat it, and we have learned a lot about how to prevent it. So why is it becoming still more common?

I have been a cardiologist for about thirty years, and during that time I have marvelled at how steady is the flow of patients with coronary artery disease. These patients are, on average older now than they were at the beginning of my career, and we are better at treating them, but about a third of them still die immediately or within a month of the first symptoms of a heart attack. And they have just kept coming to the emergency rooms. As a young cardiologist in various hospitals in Denmark, I would jot down bits of information from the ambulance driver and anyone else accompanying the patient, and we would then transfer him — it was usually a him — as quickly as possible to the relative safety of the coronary care unit. That's where we had the best equipment for treating cardiac arrest should that happen. The drugs we have now increase the chance of survival. We can also now do x-ray studies of the coronary arteries, and clots that have stopped the flow of blood can be dissolved by drugs or removed with catheters soon after symptoms begin.

Neither catheter procedures of that sort nor coronary artery by-pass surgery can prevent most heart attacks, however. That is because atherosclerosis in one part of the artery is almost always accompanied by atherosclerosis elsewhere in the artery. The catheter procedure, and the by-pass operation, removes or by-passes only one or a few of the atherosclerotic lesions of the coronary arteries. They cannot do anything about most of the atherosclerosis in these arteries.

As a young cardiologist I also began to contribute very modestly to research into the causes of coronary artery disease. That was in Copenhagen and San Francisco, and some of the details in this book reflect my Danish-American background. I now work as a professor of preventive cardiology at the University of Aarhus in Denmark. In a sense it is an easy job, because it is not difficult to prevent coronary artery disease. If you do not smoke, if you eat a mainly vegetarian diet, and if you use the muscles of your body as they were intended to be used, it is unlikely that you will be struck down by coronary artery disease before you are old. The disease should therefore be on the decline. It has in fact declined in Europe and North America, but the decline may have stopped, and in the rest of the world the disease is on the increase. Why?

The WHO provides two reasons. One is that people everywhere are living longer, because infectious diseases are on the decline. If you do not get an infection that could have killed you through diarrhoea in childhood, you survive, perhaps to die of coronary artery disease at a much greater age. That's good. Certainly no one would suggest that coronary artery disease should be prevented by promoting infections or by shooting us all on our 60th birthday, although that would in fact prevent most heart attacks.

The other reason is that people in the developing countries are taking up smoking on a large scale. That's not so good, and it identifies an agricultural context that we do not discuss very often. The big tobacco companies have, for good reasons, been the object of much recrimination, but cigarettes are made from tobacco raised by farmers. Smoking causes clots that close the coronary arteries, but clots close arteries only if the arteries have been damaged by atherosclerosis. Enter the farmer once again. Farmers raise animals, and most researchers believe that it is the meat, fat and milk from our big domesticated mammals that cause atherosclerosis.

Our health promotion efforts are directed at individuals. Don't smoke, make healthy food choices, exercise regularly, and ask your doctor to measure your blood pressure and blood cholesterol. Those effort are all well founded, but it is evident that they will not stop the advance of coronary artery disease. That is primarily because they stop short, I believe, when they get to certain societal contexts, the agricultural one in particular. Farmers raise the crops and animals that they can sell, and an important part of their net earnings is from subsidies and income supports. How much money is used to subsidize what is a political decision. I shall argue in this book that agricultural policy should be formulated within the context, not only of the adequacy of food supplies, but also within the context of the agricultural determinants of chronic diseases such as coronary artery disease. Conversely, health care policy makes little sense if there is no recognition that disease is so often the direct result of how and what we farm. Social engineering is currently not considered politically correct, but a bit of social engineering is precisely what is needed if we want to be serious about preventing coronary artery disease.

This is the age of many things including biotechnology, and as we enter the 21st century, we are given the impression that biotechnology will provide the means to prevent and cure disease. That will happen to only a very limited extent, however, despite obscenely huge investments in the life sciences. I shall try to show in this book that coronary artery disease and common conditions such as high blood pressure, high blood cholesterol and diabetes are much more complicated than the proponents of the biotechnological solution to disease would have us believe. The quality of biological and medical science has suffered, because so much of it has been based on simplistic assumptions about the relationship of genes to physiology and biochemistry. I shall argue that we must find better methods of accommodating the reality of biological complexity and diversity in future research.

Care of the sick, which is called "health care" in Newspeak, also suffers if it is based on simplistic concepts of disease. I will argue that the way we now are organizing "health care" is predicated on such simplistic concepts of disease, and that our patients are already suffering as a result. I have spent many hours of my life at morning conferences reporting, and later listening, to young physicians reporting how they have passed the night in the emergency room and the coronary care unit. The nature of those discussions has changed over the years. A generation ago the discussions were about the particularities of each patient. We still discuss those particularities, of course, but now we tend to focus on whether they are consistent with criteria for inclusion into a randomized clinical trial. The patient is usually lucky if they are. They are especially lucky if they happen to fit exactly into the mold of the trial or the quality control program designed for an idealized average patient with a common disease. Unhappily, most patients don't fit into the mold very well, and they would have been better served by physicians concerned with their particularities and with the particularities of the disease afflicting them. In this book I shall try to indicate how modifications of currently used statistical methods and quality control concepts could allow us to contemplate once again the rich detail of clinical diversity.

The latest period of political activism in Europe and the United States began in the late 1950s, and it lasted for more than 40 years. Debates and political campaigns of the period reflected the cold war as well as the real wars between the communist countries and the United States and allied countries. The debates changed, and sometimes they petered out, when the Soviet Union collapsed, partly because there was no longer any funding of political activity by intelligence agencies like the KGB.[3] More importantly, the debates changed because a vastly more complex and confusing world replaced a world that had been simply divided into camps embracing and opposing Marxism. Since 1989, we have gradually become less concerned, not only with national and international politics, but also with the politics of medicine, with the influence of industry on our universities, and with the possibilities and limitations of science. It is disturbing that young scientists, young physicians, young hospital managers, young representatives of industry, et cetera, are even less critical of increasingly intrusive managerial control of research and medicine than those of us who have entered the last years of our professional lives. That is wrong, because the conceptual underpinnings of science, health care management, industry and politics are important. In my view, they are more important than knowing the latest news about the ever so slight advantages of this, that or the other drug, even if that drug is for a disease so common that fortunes can be made by increasing the drug's share of the market by a few percentage points.

As the reader may have discerned by now, this book is less about coronary artery disease than it is about certain contexts that I believe are important for a better understanding of this disease and several others. The contexts are biological, clinical, managerial, social and historical, and each chapter is an inquiry into one or more of them. A theme common especially to the last chapters is that the balance between principle and diversity, or between Platonic idealism and Aristotelian empiricism, has been shifted too far in favor of the former, and that this imbalance is inimical to science, agriculture and clinical medicine. Here are some of the things I wish to discuss:

- When and why did coronary artery disease become quantitatively important, and are we correctly assessing current changes in occurrence of the disease? Those questions and others are addressed in Chapters 1 and 2.
- The World Health Organization prediction that coronary artery disease will lead the list of most burdensome diseases by 2020 has some fairly straightforward implications for health care policy, but in Chapter 3, I shall argue that the same prediction should also have implications for agricultural policies.
- Sometimes we allow results of scientific inquiry to guide policy decisions, sometimes we don't. Chapter 4 exploits the 20th century debate about cholesterol and heart disease as a case study of one relationship of cardiovascular science to health policy.
- How well do we know that atherosclerosis is caused by eating the meat and drinking the milk of our big domesticated mammals? In Chapter 5, I shall argue that we know this well, and that our love of milk has even been etched into our genome.
- Is coronary artery disease just the most trivial of many unfortunate consequences of modern agriculture? Chapter 6 is a brief foray into the history and future of agriculture, which is unfamiliar territory for most physicians like me. I shall draw on projections made by the Food and Agricultural Organization of the United Nations and by the International Food Policy Research Institute in Washington, D.C.

- Are we less than candid or just naïve when we ask the public to invest enormous amounts of money in working out the genetic basis of complex diseases such as coronary artery disease, when we know that the principles of Mendelian genetics almost never apply to them? Chapter 7 is an attempt at critical evaluation of the idea that knowing the genes will tell us how the body works.
- In Chapter 8, I shall argue that answering basic scientific questions in biology and epidemiology is becoming more difficult as the academic discipline of molecular biology is merging with the applied science of biotechnology, as research becomes increasingly entangled in issues of intellectual property rights, and as closer ties between universities and industry require researchers to focus on projects with commercial potential.
- In Chapter 9, I shall argue that understandable priorities in clinical medicine, re-emergence of a simple biological determinism, and, paradoxically, the emergence of evidence-based medicine, all combine to make it more difficult to understand the social, political and agricultural context of coronary artery disease.
- What tricks did statistics and classical epidemiology play on us when we, as scientists and physicians, led hospital managers to believe that the almost infinite diversity of clinical medicine could be condensed into a few categories of diseases manageable by computerized quality control programs? In Chapter 10, I shall attempt to argue that underpinning the management of our health care systems are seriously flawed concepts of such diseases as coronary artery disease.

I have already presented my credentials to the reader, and it is embarrassingly apparent that any expertise that I might have is limited to one or two of the questions just listed. The reason for writing as a single author with such serious limitations is that I have wanted to consider each question from the same bird's eye view of a larger picture. Some of the motifs of that picture are that we have had too little interest in the obvious connections between heart disease and agriculture, and that we have paid insufficient respect to the complexity and diversity of the genetics, pathophysiology and clinical aspects of this and other diseases. I believe, therefore, that we are off track in the way we think about coronary artery disease, and I doubt that I could have persuaded five other authors to share that particular preoccupation with the subject!

Others have written more comprehensively and systematically about every one of the several aspects of coronary artery disease that I shall discuss in this book. I shall refer to several of these articles, books and reports as the story develops, but the story itself is not the same as that told by others, and I hope that it will provide a perspective somewhat different from that in more comprehensive and systematic reviews.

Other diseases, moreover, could have served as well for some of the discussions in this book. Coronary artery disease is the one I know a little bit about, however, and most readers will also know enough about it to follow me into these discussions. If he or she does not, Appendix 1 provides a crash course. It is necessary to make one point here, however. Coronary heart disease is due to coronary artery disease, but the two terms are not synonymous. Coronary artery disease almost always means narrowing of the arteries that supply the heart muscle with nutrients and oxygen. Since the arteries surround the heart like a corona, or crown, they are called coronary arteries. Coronary heart disease is disease of the heart muscle due to narrowing of the coronary arteries. Coronary artery disease is more prevalent than coronary heart disease. That is because atherosclerosis, and indeed several other diseases, can affect the coronary arteries without narrowing them sufficiently to deprive the heart of oxygen and nutrients. In this book, I shall generally use the term coronary artery disease. The dictum that we are as old as our arteries is consistent with a recent redefinition of heart attack (myocardial infarction) by the major societies of cardiology in Europe and the United States.[4] The new designation, *coronary artery disease with heart attack*, emphasizes the dependency of coronary heart disease on coronary artery disease.

Atherosclerosis and clotting (thrombosis), and thereby most cases of coronary artery disease and coronary heart disease, are preventable. Atherosclerosis is less likely to develop if one eats a diet rich in fruits, vegetables, whole grain and fish. A diet of this kind works not only by lowering concentrations of cholesterol in blood. It also cools off the artery wall by combating inflammation, and it makes clotting of blood less likely. Blood clotting is also less likely to occur if one does not smoke. Diabetes and high blood pressure increase the risk of coronary artery disease, and both conditions develop more readily in fat people. Avoiding obesity is therefore yet another way to avoid coronary artery disease.

All of this can be done without any help at all from our enormous health care systems. An apple a day keeps the doctor away. At the turn of the century, however, there were substantial advances in the treatment of patients with coronary artery disease and coronary heart disease. Therapy with drugs and surgery is the subject of countless conferences, articles and books. Surgery to by-pass narrow parts of coronary arteries really does lessen symptoms, and in some patients it probably improves prognosis. The same applies to dilation of narrow parts by small balloons and little stents, inserted by cardiologists with long, thin catheters threaded through the arteries from the groin. Such procedures lessen chest pain, and they can dislodge the clots that have closed the arteries in very ill patients. Moreover, drugs to lower blood pressure, blood cholesterol or heart rate as well as drugs to dilate arteries or inhibit clotting of blood really do alleviate symptoms and lessen the risk of heart attacks. I've spent much of my life helping patients with treatment of this kind, especially with drugs. All of these advances are exciting, and in the economically developed countries there is an enormous medico-industrial complex in place to exploit them.

They are not the main subject of this book, however. Although I have tried to ensure that the information I give is up to date, the book is not a review of the literature. It has the wider and mostly less technical focus that I have tried to sketch by these introductory remarks. Biologists will find that the biology is very elementary, and cardiologists will find that the cardiology is similarly elementary. The same pertains to administrators, nurses, economists, farmers, agronomists, historians, statisticians, technicians, geneticists and people entirely without obvious expertise in the subject matters touched upon in this book. For that very reason, however, I hope that experts and non-experts alike will be encouraged to think about the larger context of diseases such as coronary artery disease.

Let us begin by seeing what we know about when and why coronary artery disease turned up in human history in the first place. Always look back before changing lanes.

Chapter 1

Coronary Artery Disease Before 1920

We do not know when atherosclerosis of the coronary arteries first caused one of our ancestors to clutch his chest in pain. It must have been several thousand years ago, but we do not know how often it happened before the early 20th century. As that century opened, the disease was probably not very common, and most physicians knew almost nothing about it. By the middle of the 20th century it had become epidemic in economically developed counties, and despite a later decline in those countries, the World Health Organization estimates that by 2020 it will be the single most burdensome disease to the health systems of the world.

Everyone now knows something about coronary heart disease. In some countries, even school children are taught cardiac resuscitation. Why was the disease almost unknown before 1900, and how did it become so common and obvious in the developed countries by the mid-20th century? How can we prevent it from spreading to the developing countries? And finally, if we can't stop spreading the disease, why can't we?

These questions are all based on an assumption that some people have found contentious. That coronary artery disease was rare in the past and common now is the dominant point of view, but it is not necessarily correct. Critics of that view have in fact called "*the concept of an epidemic of heart disease . . . a 20th century myth*." The crux of that argument is that aging of populations accounts, by and large, for the apparent increase in disease occurrence.[1] It has, in fact, been surprisingly difficult to work out whether the disease is a newcomer or whether it has always been with us. Public health efforts and preventive cardiology make a lot of sense if the disease is a newcomer. They make less sense if it just part of the human condition. As we shall see later, the demographic explanation is certain to be partially correct, but it is not tenable as a complete explanation. It has nevertheless been important, because it has justified doing little or nothing to prevent the disease.

Like many of the other diseases of "internal medicine", coronary artery disease does not lend itself well to historical inquiry. It causes no specific symptoms. There are many other reasons for clutching one's chest in real or apparent pain, and other diseases kill suddenly. Therefore, the history of diseases such as coronary heart disease cannot be written apart from the history of the medical disciplines that allow us to detect them.

This problem does not pertain to all diseases. We know quite a lot about the history of some infectious diseases like Bubonic Plague. In the middle of the 14th century the Plague killed about 25 million people in Europe, a quarter of the population. We now know that Plague is due to the bacterium, yersinia pestis, even though bacteriology did not appear on the scene until the 19th century. The disease identified itself by a swelling of the lymph nodes in the neck, groin or armpit, bleeding into the skin and sometimes by rapidly fatal pneumonia, and there is no doubt that the Black Death of 14th century Europe was Bubonic Plague. Everyone knew about it: *"A plague o' both your houses!"*

Our ancestors were also familiar with cancer. In fact, an old Danish oath, *"kræftæideme,"* means *"may cancer eat me"* (if what I'm telling you is not true). Coronary heart disease is altogether a different matter, not at all like the Black Death, despite what the European Society of Cardiology has to say about it. I know not one proper oath invoking heart attacks.

Paleopathology

The history of any disease and the history of the medical disciplines employed in studying it are obviously not the same thing. Coronary artery disease would or would not have been there, irrespective of whether pathology, medicine or cardiology had been there to detect it. The two kinds of history, that of the object and that of the way to look at the object, are nevertheless intertwined. The only way to look at the early history of coronary artery disease is by paleopathology and the examination of scant historical records. In the following, I shall draw substantially on the history of the disease by J. O. Leibowitz of the Hebrew University in Jerusalem.[2]

Paleopathology is the study of disease in animals or humans who died a long time ago. In the first decades of the 20th century, paleopathological studies of Egyptian mummies demonstrated unequivocal atherosclerosis of the aorta and probable atherosclerosis of smaller arteries (the aorta is the body's main artery). The coronary arteries were not the object of early studies, but in 1931 the coronary arteries of a female mummy from the 21st dynasty (about 1,000 B.C.) showed *"marked fibrous thickening, chiefly of the intima, with calcification."* The intima is the innermost layer of the artery, and the changes described in the study were almost certainly due to atherosclerosis. The woman was approximately 50 years old when she died. She also had diseases of the lungs and kidneys, and the disease of her coronary arteries was not necessarily the cause of her death.

In his recent book, Darwin R. Labarthe remarks that although these paleopathological studies do "not establish that atherosclerosis was epidemic in ancient times, as it has become more recently; it can be presumed that those whose remains were so carefully prepared for burial were members of particularly affluent, and possibly high-risk strata of those early societies".[3] Labarthe is right, but we can add that paleopathology is not our only way to probe disease occurrence in ancient Egypt.

Historical Records

Rare or not, coronary artery disease must have caused symptoms in some of the ancient Egyptians. Whether the Egyptian physicians recognized those symptoms as being related to disease of the heart cannot be known with certainty, but one passage in the

Ebers Papyrus from Thebes, dating back to about 1550 B.C., suggests that possibility. Leibowitz quotes it in the following way:

> When you examine a man for illness in his cardia, he has pains in his arm, in his breast, on the side of his cardia; it is said thereof: this is the . . . illness. Then you shall say thereof: it is something which entered his mouth; it is death which approaches him. Then you shall prepare for him stimulating herbal remedies: fruits of pea, bryony [and other vegetable remedies], let them be boiled in fat . . . and be drunk by the man. Put then your bended hand on him, until the arm gets well and free of pains. Then you shall say: this illness has descended to the rectum, to the anus. The remedy shall not then be repeated.

Leibowitz writes that the supposed connection between a cardiac condition and the rectum is typical of Egyptian medicine, a notion of elimination of noxious substances. The term cardia can signify the heart as well as the stomach. The context in this passage suggests that it is the former, and the man's affliction had the classical hallmarks of angina pectoris: the attack was transitory ("*until the arm gets well and free of pains*"), it had the right topography ("*pains in his arm, in his breast, on the side of the cardia*"), and the patient was terrified by a feeling of impending death ("*it is death which approaches him*"). If this interpretation of the Ebers Papyrus is correct, it suggests that angina pectoris was not extremely rare in ancient Egypt. It was at least common enough to be part of what physicians taught their students. It is also the first recorded attempt to explain what causes angina pectoris. More than 3,000 years would elapse before someone came up with a better explanation.

The writings of Hippocrates (5th century B.C.), Galen (2nd century A.D.), the Talmud, as well as writings from Byzantium and medieval Europe, do not contain any clear indications of knowledge of coronary artery disease. In medieval Europe, though, laymen described calamities likely to have been fatal heart attacks. The sudden death of the Count de Foix in 1392 was described in the following way by a contemporary:

> The day he died, he had all the forenoon been hunting a bear. The weather was marvellously hot, even for the month of August. In the evening [at the inn] he called for water to wash and stretched out his hands; but no sooner had his fingers . . . touched the cold water, than he changed colour, from an oppression at his heart, and, his legs failing him, fell back on his seat, exclaiming, "I am a dead man: Lord God, have mercy on me!" He never spoke after this, though he did not immediately die, but sufferered great pain . . . In less than half an hour he was dead, having surrendered his soul very quietly.

The heat of the day, the strenuous hunt, the touching of the cold water, the oppression of the "heart" and the count's realization that he was dying are all consistent with a myocardial infarction. No one could know that then for sure, but in the 14th century things had begun to change. The authorities in Bologna permitted dissections of human bodies, beginning the era of modern medicine. Later the anatomical studies of Leonardo da Vinci (1452–1519) included the coronary arteries. During the next $2\frac{1}{2}$ centuries, physicans described, here and there, patients who could well have had the disease. The term angina pectoris was first used in 1772 by the British physician William Heberden (1710–1801) when he wrote one of the passages of medical history most often quoted in textbooks and pharmaceutical advertisements:

> There is a disorder of the breast . . . The seat of it, and sense of strangling and anxiety, with which it is attended, may make it not improperly be called angina pectoris. Those, who are afflicted with it, are ceased [sic!] while they are walking and most particularly when they walk soon after eating, with a painful and most disagreeable sensation in the breast, which seems as it would take their breath away, if it were to increase or to continue; the moment they stand still, all this uneasiness vanishes.

Although Heberden did not explicitly connect these symptoms with coronary artery disease, that connection was made only a few years later by his friend and colleague, Edward Jenner (1749–1823). Jenner did this in a letter that he wrote to Heberden in 1776. In the letter he describes his concern for his patient, John Hunter.[4]

> When you are acquainted with my motives, I presume you will pardon the liberty I take in addressing you. I am prompted to it from a knowledge of the mutual regard that subsists between you and my worthy friend Mr. Hunter. When I had the pleasure of seeing him at Bath last autumn I thought he was affected with many symptoms of the angina pectoris. The dissections (as far as I have seen) of those who have died of it throw little light upon the subject. Though, in the course of my practice, I have seen many fall victims to this dreadful disease, yet I have only had two opportunities of an examination after death. In the first of these I found no material disease of the heart, except that the coronary artery appeared thickened.
>
> As no notice had been taken of such a circumstance by anybody who had written on the subject, I concluded that we must still seek for other causes as productive of the disease; but, about three weeks ago, Mr. Paytherus, a surgeon at Ross, in Herefordshire, desired me to examine with him the heart of a person who had died of the angina pectoris a few days before. Here we found the same appearance of the coronary arteries as in the former case. But what I had taken to be an ossification of the vessel itself, Mr. P. discovered to be a kind of firm, fleshy tube, formed within the vessel, with a considerable quantity of ossific matter dispersed irregularly through it. This tube did not appear to have any vascular connection with the coats of the artery, but seemed to lie merely in simple contact with it.
>
> As the heart, I believe, in every subject that has died of the angina pectoris, has been found extremely loaded with fat, and as these vessels lie quite concealed in that substance, is it possible this appearance may have been overlooked? The importance of the coronaries, and how much the heart must suffer from their not being able to duly perform their functions (we can not be surprised at the painful spasms), is a subject I

need not enlarge upon, therefore shall just remark that it is possible that all the symptoms may arise from this one circumstance.

As I frequently write to Mr. H. I have been some time in hesitation respecting the propriety of communicating the matter to him, and should be exceedingly thankful to you, sir, for your advice upon the subject. Should it be admitted that this is the cause of the disease, I fear the medical world may seek in vain for a remedy, and I am fearful (if Mr. Hunter should admit this to be the cause of the disease) that it may deprive him of the hopes of a recovery.

John Hunter survived until 1793. A surgeon and physiologist, he was Edward Jenner's friend and mentor in medicine, probably explaining the level of concern expressed in this letter. John Hunter founded pathological anatomy in England, made several important contributions to surgery, and was a proponent of experimentation. He contracted syphilis by inoculating himself in an attempt to show that syphilis and gonorrhoea are manifestations of the same disease, and his angina pectoris was not necessarily due to atherosclerosis. It could have been due to syphilitic disease of the aorta or the coronary arteries.

Jenner's letter to Heberden briefly unites for medical history three great English physicians of the 18th century. Jenner's main contribution to medicine was his discovery and promotion of vaccination against smallpox. As is evident from this letter, however, he also clearly made the connection between angina pectoris and disease of the coronary arteries, and the *"fleshy tube ... with ... a considerable quantity of ossific matter dispersed irregularly throughout it"* is very likely to have been atherosclerosis. Nevertheless, nearly a century and a half would pass before the connection between angina pectoris and disease of the coronary arteries was generally known and accepted by the medical profession.

The 19th century saw the studies leading to the essentials of modern concepts of atherosclerosis and thrombosis. Rudolf Virchov (1821–1902), especially, although not much interested in the coronary arteries,[2] developed the fundamental concepts of the way blood clots are made and how they can travel through the blood vessels to other parts of the body (thrombosis and embolism). He was the dominant figure in the great era of German biomedical research for half a century,[5] and, more than anyone else, he showed that diseases had to be understood in terms of cell theory. Cells were to the 19th century what molecules became to the 20th. The study of cells required good microscopes, and they became widely available in mid-century, especially in Germany, where Carl Zeiss set up a workshop in Jena in 1846. Virchow and his many pupils established the importance of cells in cancer, inflammation and thrombosis. By1882, the participation of white blood cells and especially of blood platelets in thrombosis had been worked out,[6] and at the beginning of the 21st century, we still understand thrombosis largely as Virchow did.

One of the central concepts of research in atherosclerosis during the last two decades of the 20th century has been a particular vulnerability of the inflamed atherosclerotic plaques. We shall develop this concept fully a little later, but let us touch upon it here. The two main components of atherosclerosis are a pocket of soft material inside a capsule of hard fibrous tissue. The soft material is the *"athere,"* a Greek word for porridge, and the hard fibrous tissue is the sclerotic part of the disease. *"Skleros"* is the Greek word for *"hard."* The porridge has the consistency of toothpaste. If the capsule is inflamed, it can weaken and rupture so that the porridge oozes into the blood. When that happens, blood forms a thrombus, and the artery can be closed off rapidly and completely.

Thrombosis and inflammation are important from an epidemiological point of view, because both can come and go rapidly, like a cold or a rash. If inflammation of the artery wall affected many people, its coming and going could in part explain the rise and fall of atherosclerotic and thrombotic disease in the 20th century. It is unlikely to be a new phenomenon, however, because we can be almost certain that it occurred at least occasionally in the 19th century. We know that, for example, from an autopsy which was reported to a meeting of a Danish medical society in March of 1844. The report concerned the death of Bertel Thorvaldsen.

Thorvaldsen was a sculptor, and he was world-famous for his neo-classicist art, especially in his own country of Denmark. He was particularly world-famous in Copenhagen, and in his lifetime the city built a museum for his sculptures right next to the Castle of Copenhagen, which now houses Parliament. In 1844, at the age of 75, he had for some time suffered from oppression of the chest. As a celebrity, several physicians tended to him, very much in competition with each other. None of them seemed to know more about the causes of oppression of the chest than did their predecessors in ancient Egypt, however. Thorvaldsen also suffered from osteomyelitis, a bacterial infection of the bone marrow. One of his physicians ascribed the chest pains to a closing of a fistula of the leg through which pus from the marrow of the bone had been emptied onto the skin surface. Needless to say, the closing of the fistula had been performed by this particular physician's competitor. The idea that the oppression of the chest was due to the accumulation of pus was essentially the same as the thinking apparent from the Ebers Papyrus: that angina pectoris could be relieved by the elimination of noxious substances from the body. The only difference was the orifice of exit.

When out walking Thorvaldsen had often said to his servant, "Let us stop for just a little while." He would then press his hand to his heart and say, "This chest will be my death." On the last day of his life, he dined with some good friends including Hans Christian Andersen, the story teller. He then walked the short distance from Kronprinsessegade to the Royal Theater, where he arrived slightly late, after the overture to Ferdinand Ries' 6th symphony had begun. Immediately after taking his seat, he collapsed and died. The orchestra finished the overture, and physicians in the audience did a venesection. It was of no avail.

An autopsy was performed in Thorvaldsen's home and reported two days after his death at a medical society meeting. Large parts of the aorta were atherosclerotic. It was calcified, and there was a lot of ulceration. Rupture of atherosclerotic plaques had evidently taken place several times during the recent past, and both of the coronary arteries were afflicted in the same way. In a part of the left coronary artery there were *"several atheromatous plaques, one of which quite clearly had ulcerated, pouring the atheromatous mass into the arterial lumen"*.[7]

Thus, Thorvaldsen had died of a rupture of an atherosclerotic plaque in a coronary artery, and the autopsy findings were the same as those we see now at the beginning of the 21st century. We know now that rupture is almost always due to inflammation, so there can be little doubt that Bertel Thorvaldsen's coronary arteries were inflamed, and it is not likely that he was the only person to have been so afflicted in the 1840s.

In his 1897 lectures on angina pectoris,[4] the Canadian-American physician, William Osler (1849–1919), wrote that sufferers of angina pectoris often die suddenly.

> Anatomically it has been shown that a lesion of the coronary arteries is almost invariably present — either extensive arteriosclerosis, embolism, thrombosis, or in rare instances the bursting of a small atheromatous abscess in one vessel, such as killed the celebrated sculptor Thorwaldsen. An explanation of the awful suddenness — "Life struck sharp on Death" — is probably to be found in the arrest of the heart in fibrillary contraction, such as takes place experimentally in animals after ligation of a coronary artery.

We know now that the *"bursting of . . . (an) abscess"* is not rare, but Osler's description of the connection between angina pectoris, disease of the coronary arteries and sudden death is quite clear, and he had already described it well in his great textbook of medicine, published in 1892 and *"designed for the use of practitioners and students of medicine"*.[8]

Nevertheless, it fell to the American, James B. Herrick (1861–1954), to establish that connection to the satisfaction of the medical community. Herrick is perhaps best known for the first description of sickle cell anaemia, but he also crusaded to convince physicians of the importance of coronary artery disease. He gave two papers about the subject, one in 1912 and the other in 1918. The first paper, published in the *Journal of the American Medical Association*, was a well written and complete description of the clinical features of coronary artery disease and myocardial infarction,[9] but it had no effect on physicians. In his autobiography he wrote:[2]

> The publication aroused no interest. It fell like a dud. Recognizing the radical nature of the view I held . . . I doggedly kept at the subject, doing what I called "missionary work". I hammered away at the topic. When in 1918 I showed lantern slides and electrocardiograms [of coronary obstruction], physicians in America and later Europe woke up [to the diagnosis which was] later to become a household word translated by the layman into "heart attack."

Thus, although atherosclerosis and coronary artery disease have been with us, off and on, for thousands of years, we can be quite sure that as late as 1920 understanding of the causes and mechanisms of the disease was rudimentary, most physicians were only beginning to accept the disease as clinically important, and almost none of them knew how to diagnose it. All of this has, in turn, implications for our interpretation of the data on which we base our concepts of the epidemic of coronary heart disease in the 20th century.

Chapter 2

Coronary Artery Disease 1920–2000

In 1920, the diseases of the heart most familiar to physicians were those due to infections. Bacteria could infect the valves of the heart and cause death within a matter of days or weeks. More commonly, streptococci in the throat could damage the heart indirectly, by causing rheumatic fever, a low-intensity immunological inflammation, in particular of the joints. Within a short time it could also inflame and weaken the heart muscle, and if the patient survived that attack, it could in the longer term destroy the valves of the heart.

Physicians had less first-hand experience with patients with coronary artery disease, and, as we saw in the first chapter, a graduate of an American or European medical school in 1920 did not know a lot about it. By the end of his career as a physician, however, halfway through the period covered in this chapter, coronary artery disease would have replaced rheumatic heart disease as a major cause of death. By 2000, "heart attack" had not only been a household word for more than half a century; the fat and cholesterol content of most foods sold in American supermarkets was given on the package, the connection between smoking and this disease and others had become abundantly clear, and a huge medico-industrial complex was in place in all wealthy countries to diagnose, treat and organize a steady stream of patients with coronary artery disease.

The big tobacco companies, and with them the small tobacco farmers, had begun to suffer setbacks in the American court system by the end of the 20th century, but the connection to the rest of agriculture stopped at the level of consumer choices of food products. Agricultural policy remained outside the realm of explicit medical debate, even though physicians knew that coronary artery disease had connections with the cultural values derived from our past as agriculturalists. The debate about the causes of coronary artery disease had virtually died out by the end of the century, not because it had been fundamentally resolved, but almost no one seemed truly interested in eradication. The resourceful could usually avoid the disease, and for the less resourceful or the genetically disadvantaged there were increasingly effective and sophisticated pharmacological and surgical treatments.

In mid-century, however, that understanding was still a long way off. The tobacco, meat and dairy industries felt threatened by the emergence of coronary artery disease as a public health issue, and it was still legitimate to puzzle about what caused it, and to challenge the idea that it had anything to do with the way of modern life. If one could argue that the disease had always been with us, if only we lived long enough, then agriculture would be exonerated and diagnosis and treatment of the disease could be institutionalized. On the other hand, if the disease had been more recently visited upon us, then the agent of visitation should be identified and removed, and physicians should prepare to look for something else to do. The core question was therefore whether the disease was on the rise or whether it wasn't, and the core criterion in answering that question was incidence of disease.

Establishing That There Has Been a Rise and Fall of Coronary Artery Disease in Developed Countries

Apparently a dry, technical term, incidence of disease can cause a lot of excitement and heated discourse. Incidence is the frequency of an occurrence of some kind. In medical epidemiology it means the number of new cases of a disease occurring in a population of specified size and sometimes of specified age within a specified period of time. Changes in disease incidence have profound implications for public health policies.

Incidence data based on the coding of death certificates for cause of death became available after 1900.[1] During the first two decades of the 20th century, coronary artery disease caused only about 7 annual deaths/100,000 people in the United States. There was little fluctuation in these data from year to year, but in 1920, the disease apparently took off. During the next decades it increased very sharply until it leveled off and topped in the 1960s. At that time it caused more than 300 deaths annually/100,000 Americans. These data are not adjusted for age, and changes in the age distribution within the population therefore account for part of the rise, but the rise in rates of death due to heart disease remain after taking age into account. Since deaths due to rheumatic heart disease are included in these data, and since rheumatic heart almost disappeared during this period, the rise in deaths due to coronary artery disease is actually an underestimate.

After 1968, rates of death by coronary artery disease dropped steadily until the end of the century, when they tended to stabilize and even increase once again. Similar trends have been seen elsewhere, first in Europe, later in other parts of the world. In some countries, e.g. Finland, temporal changes of this kind have been even more dramatic. Adjustment of the data for age is also important here. Because of aging populations, it is only the age-adjusted rates of death by coronary artery disease that have declined in the developed countries.

The age-adjusted rates are the ones of primary interest when we want to understand the causes of the disease. In contrast, rates of disease, adjusted for age as well as not adjusted for age, are of interest for the WHO and others involved in planning health care. This is a crucial point, and it is easy to understand when you think about it. If we prevent the disease in most people in middle age, and if our treatment of people at any age is so good that they don't die right away, then more people will survive to get the disease and succumb to it at a later age. Successful treatment of coronary artery disease (preventing deaths) can therefore, paradoxically, increase the number of people who have the disease.

There are even more important reasons why populations in the developed countries, and soon in the developing countries, are on average getting older. They include better standards of hygiene and better treatment of infectious diseases. They also contribute to an expansion of the number of people who have coronary artery disease.

On top of the ground swell of (age adjusted rates of) coronary artery disease during the 20th century have been smaller waves and wavelets. Brief fluctuations occurred during World War II when national statistics showed that deaths due to "arteriosclerosis", including coronary artery disease, continued to rise in the U.S. and were stable in Denmark, but that they fell in Sweden, Norway and Finland from 1940 to 1945.[2,3] Hagvin Malmros related these changes to the availability of dietary fat, which declined in Sweden, Norway and Finland but was stable in the USA and Denmark. No German national statistics from the war years were available, but hospital statistics indicated that the disease virtually did not occur in the immediate post-war period, 1945–1948, when undernutrition was widespread.[4]

A Dutch study of temporal changes in death rates in families with familial hypercholesterolemia extends the concept that coronary artery disease really did increase markedly at the beginning of the 20th century, reached a peak in mid-century and then declined.[5,6] The study was small, but a particular feature of the persons studied enabled the investigators to ascertain changes in rates of death almost certainly due to coronary artery disease over a longer period of time than that possible in studies of the general population. It was a look into the epidemiology of coronary artery disease from the beginning of the 19th century.

Familial hypercholesterolemia is usually due to a mutation in a gene that determines how quickly cholesterol can be removed from the blood stream. In family members with the mutation, cholesterol concentrations in blood are high, and on average they die of coronary artery disease many years before other people if they are not treated. Half of the genetically related persons in such a family have the mutation in one of their two genes for a certain protein called the LDL receptor. If a death certificate at the beginning of the 19th century shows, for example, that a person in such a family died at the age of 30 or 40, then it is very likely that the death was due to coronary artery disease.

The Dutch investigators exploited excellent public records to ascertain ages at death in 250 members of a family with the same mutation in the gene for the LDL receptor. Between 1830 and 1989, death rates (age-adjusted) in this family changed markedly. In the middle of the 19th century, they were actually lower than in the general population, but they had apparently increased by 1870, and they were significantly higher than rates in the general population during the 20th century, peaking in mid-century (1935–1964).

The only possible explanation for these findings is that the age at which family members with the mutation succumbed to coronary artery disease began to fall during the last decades of the 19th century, and that they hit bottom, in the middle of the 20th century. They died quite young. This was much too short a time period for any change in the genes to have occurred. It could only mean that important environmental changes had taken place. This fits in with results of other studies showing that risk of coronary artery disease increases disproportionately in people with familial hypercholesterolemia when risk factors such as smoking and unhealthy diets become common in the population. Like miners' canaries, members of these families are particularly sensitive to changes in the environment. Methodologically independent of the approach of the large population studies, the Dutch study therefore suggests that coronary artery disease was already becoming more common in the last 2–3 decades of the 19th century.

Taken together, these data are consistent with a very close association of the disease with industrialization and urbanization, which was well advanced in the United States and in western Europe, Great Britain especially, by the end of the 19th century.[7] One way to understand coronary artery disease is, in fact, to consider it one of the many consequences of industrialization and urbanization. Indeed, Salim Yusuf and his colleagues consider the disease a consequence of our failure to adapt intelligently to life as city dwellers.[8]

It was only when it also became possible on a wide scale to ascertain the disease in the general population that public records and population studies began to reflect what was really going on. It is now easy to understand the sharp increase in the rates of the disease from 1920 onwards: it was due to the quite sudden recognition of a disease that was already on the increase. The observations only had to catch up with reality.

What made it possible to identify the disease on a wider scale? Diagnosis was not as easy as it might seem at the present time. Many other diseases cause chest pain, and without the electrocardiogram no physician would, even now, venture making a diagnosis that implies treatment with drugs to dissolve blood clots or combat irregularities of heart rhythm. He would probably be taken to court if he did, because some of these treatments are risky, and the risk is worthwhile only if the diagnosis is fairly certain.

Measurement of the electrical activity of the heart became possible with Willem Einthoven's invention in 1903 of a string galvanometer for electrocardiography. Versions of the electrocardiograph suitable for clinical work became available only in the 1920s, however, and it took the 1920s and the 1930s to identify the abnormalities in electrocardiographic recordings that would make it easy for physicians to see whether a patient had a myocardial infarction. The other essential for the diagnosis of myocardial infarction was some sort of measurement of changes in the cellular or chemical components of blood. Cellular indicators of myocardial infarction were high numbers of white blood cells or an abnormal tendency of red blood cells to settle at the bottom of a test tube. These laboratory analyses were in use before World War II, but the modern era of biochemical markers did not open until the 1950s. That happened when it became easy to measure transaminases in blood. Transaminases are enzymes that belong inside cells. If cells die, as they do in heart muscle when a coronary artery is closed off, the enzymes leak into the blood stream in much greater quantities than usual.

Technology of this sort was one of the prerequisites for several large epidemiological studies to find the causes of and to monitor the course of the disease. We shall return to the question of causes later and concentrate here on the course of the disease. In the 1960s it seemed apparent that coronary artery disease was again declining in the United States, but the decline had no obvious explanation. As a result of a conference on *The Decline in Coronary Artery Disease Mortality,* held in 1978, a large international project (MONICA) was instigated in order to answer the question as to whether the reported declines were genuine. If they were genuine, the second question was how much of the decline could be attributed to improved survival rather than to declining event rates? In other words, was the decline due to better treatment (lower case fatality) or had the disease again become less common (lower incidence)? The question of the relative importance of case fatality rates and incidence rates has implications for balancing investments in medical or surgical therapy against investments in environmental changes including public health measures. The MONICA project was, metaphorically speaking, designed to get to the heart of the matter: was cardiovascular disease, including coronary artery disease, stable or was it changing?

MONICA is an acronym for "*moni*toring trends and determinants in *ca*rdiovascular disease". The MONICA project, executed under the auspices of the WHO, was one of many large epidemiological studies of the 20th century. It registered about 166,000 fatal and non-fatal heart attacks that had occurred in 37 different population groups in 21 different countries over a period of approximately 10 years between the early 1980s and the early 1990s. The people to be followed were between 35 and 64 years old, and the countries selected for study were those in which declines in rates of disease were thought to have occurred. They were therefore not representative of the world. There were 11 countries in western Europe, 2 countries in North America (USA and Canada), Australia and New Zealand, and 5 former socialist countries of eastern Europe including Russia. China also participated, but there were no other Asian countries, and there were no countries in Africa or South America.

The results were published in 1999.[9] The MONICA death rates tended to be higher than the official mortality rates, but on the basis of both sets of data, the study could answer "yes" to the first question of the 1978 conference. The declines in coronary heart disease rates noted in the USA and other developed countries were genuine, in part because they were so large and consistent that no competing causes of death were large enough to have absorbed them. In countries with a decline, the average annual rates of decline were 4.6% in men and 3.7% in women. Rates did not decline in all countries, however. With the exception of Yugoslavia, mortality rates increased in all the former socialist countries of eastern Europe including Russia; they also increased in China. On average, annual rates of increase were 1.7% in men and 1.9% in women.

The second question of the 1978 conference could also be answered clearly. In countries experiencing a decline in coronary death rates, two thirds of the decline could be ascribed to lower incidence and one third to lower case fatality. In other words, the fact that fewer people were getting the disease in the first place was twice as important as better survival once you had the disease. The overall death rate is related to incidence and case fatality rates in the following way: the number of people dying of the disease equals the number who get the disease in the first place multiplied by the fraction who die of the disease.

$$\text{coronary death rate} = \text{incidence} \times \text{case fatality}$$

With units, the equation looks like this:

$$\text{deaths/population} = \text{coronary events/population} \times \text{deaths/coronary event}$$

The authors of the MONICA report wrote that "*despite substantial contributions from changing survival, the main determinant of the decline in CHD mortality is whatever drives the changing coronary-event rates"*. This conclusion implies that citizens of our various countries would benefit more from preventive than from therapeutic efforts. They would in fact benefit twice as much. But could that conclusion be somehow biased so that any policy based on it would be distorted?

The authors identified two sources of bias in ascertaining case fatality rates in the former socialist countries and in the economically more developed countries. They were not of the same kind. In the former socialist countries, the contributions of increasing incidence and increasing case fatalities to the increase in coronary death rates were calculated to be about equal. One possible explanation for increasing case fatality rates in these countries could have been deteriorating standards of treatment, but the authors suggested a more plausible explanation: *"Pressures to misuse coronary diagnoses to conceal increasing drug-related or alcohol-related deaths would lead to increases in apparent case fatality"*. In other words, passing off a death which is really due to alcoholism as one due to a heart attack contributes to the impression that heart attacks are more often fatal, because there is probably no corresponding inclination to pass off a non-fatal binge as a non-fatal heart attack. If the reader will refer to the equation just given, it is easy to see that any overestimation of the case fatality rates means that the contribution of an increase in incidence to increasing coronary death rates will be correspondingly underestimated.

In ascertaining rates of case fatality in the developed countries, there could have been a reverse problem. The authors wrote that *"better identification of minor, otherwise silent infarction, better access to health care, more intensive use of sensitive tests, and rejection of doubtful deaths would lower it"*. This situation is in fact very common in hospitals in the developed world. In explaining decreasing coronary death rates, it follows that overestimation of the fall in case fatality will cause a fall in incidence to be underestimated. The true contribution of better treatment to the drop in coronary mortality in the developed countries from the early 1980s to the early 1990s may therefore have been less than a third.

To the extent that policies of public health are based on scientific evidence, bias in interpretation of scientific data will distort policy. In the former socialist countries, real but less presentable causes of deterioration of public health were perhaps neglected. In the developed countries, treatment was perhaps accorded more emphasis than it deserved. In both cases, the MONICA Project might have underestimated changes in incidence, i.e. the rates at which people get the disease in the first place. The relative importance of prevention and treatment is therefore likely to be even more in favor of prevention than was estimated by the MONICA Project.

Now let us for a moment focus on the most important implication of the studies that we have discussed so far in this chapter. It is that coronary artery disease in the developed countries really did become much more prevalent by the time the 20th century opened, and that it peaked shortly after mid-century. Given the nature of the disease, it is almost certain that a similar historical trend would apply to other atherosclerotic disease, and, in fact, a recent study of secular trends in stroke in England and Wales shows that the occurrence of strokes due to clots (ischemic stroke) but not bleedings (hemorrhagic stroke) closely matches the rise and fall of coronary artery disease.[1]

Because these diseases have affected so many people, the changes in the rates of occurrence were momentous, but because they also happened slowly, they were at the same time not very obvious at all.

Understanding the Rise and Fall of Coronary Artery Disease

The slowness of the appearance and disappearance of the disease not only made it difficult to see that they were occurring. It also made it difficult to work out what caused them. One piece of understanding was clear from the beginning: the changes in the incidence of coronary artery disease must have been due to changes in the environment. The rise and fall of coronary artery disease in the 20th century may have been too slow for the human brain to appreciate it very easily, but the process occurred far too quickly to be due to any conceivable change in the human genome.

Such environmental changes could be medical, but most of them are more likely to be outside the realm of medicine, simply because most deaths due to coronary artery disease still occur outside hospitals,[11,12] and because systematic screening of populations for high risk patients and treatment of such patients have not been done to any appreciable extent in any country. But which environmental changes outside the realm of medicine? Working that out has been one of the great challenges of medical epidemiology, and countless articles have been written about it, not only in medical journals but also in serious as well as more frivolous publications from the lay press.

Hundreds of environmental factors are more or less closely associated with occurrence of the disease, and I shall discuss some of them in later chapters, especially those related to agriculture. Some of them are societal, such as industrialization, organization of transport systems, and the provision of tobacco, and certain foods by agriculture. Others are subject to choices that can be made by individuals, such as what and how much to eat, whether or not to take a run, take a hike, use the bike or car, and whether or not to smoke the next cigarette. The list of dietary factors is particularly long. In the remainder of this chapter, however, I want to focus on two aspects of the disease bearing on our understanding of how it changes over time. One is the temporal relationship of changes in risk factors to changes in disease rates: the disease lags substantially behind the appearance of risk factors. That aspect is central to the 20th century debate about what to do, or whether to do anything, to prevent the disease. Much confusion could have been avoided had we in mid-century had a better understanding of the importance of time lag.

The other is our turn-of-the-century understanding of the pathology of the disease as it appears on autopsy, under the microscope and in physiological and molecular biology laboratories. It is in that pathology that we now seem to have identified the properties of the disease that have allowed it to be transformed, within a human life-time or two, from a rare to a common disease.

Time Lag

Changes in rates of coronary heart disease have not always had the expected close relationships to fluctuations in risk factors, and as late as 1980 those temporal relationships remained elusive. In his history of the epidemic of the disease, Stallones wrote that *"hypertension does not fit the trend of the mortality from ischemic heart disease at all; physical activity fits only the rising curve, serum cholesterol fits only the falling curve and only cigarette smoking fits both. In no case is the fit as precise as one would like. This raises doubt that any of the factors is a fully satisfactory explanation for the variation in mortality."* [1]

You will come down with the flu a few days after exposure, and in fact you sometimes know exactly who gave it to you. With one exception, none of the risk factors for coronary heart disease causes disease so quickly as to be obvious. The exception is fortunately so rare that very few physicians have ever seen it. Children younger than five years old can die of coronary artery disease if they have inherited two mutated genes rather than just one mutated gene for familial hypercholesterolemia (homozygosity). Since they have extensive deposits of cholesterol, not only in their arteries but also in their skin and tendons, the connection between coronary disease and cholesterol is obvious.

Most people with coronary artery disease have never had concentrations of cholesterol in their blood close to those of children with homozygous familial hypercholesterolemia, and the garden variety of atherosclerosis takes many years to become mature and ready to kill. On average 60% of the surface area of the large arteries has been transmogrified by advanced atherosclerosis by the time symptoms first appear to cut off life or make it miserable.[13,14] The implication is that the clinical phase of the disease lags way behind the initial phases.

Not all population studies can tell us about time lag. Since cross-sectional studies are performed at one point in time, they tell us nothing about temporal relationships, but time lag becomes apparent from results of longitudinal studies lasting many years. The importance of time lag for our understanding of the causes of coronary artery disease emerged clearly from an analysis by two English epidemiologists of the relationship of coronary disease mortality in 20 countries, not only to past and present concentrations of cholesterol in blood, but also to past and present consumption of animal fats.[15]

Coronary artery disease death rates in 1992 were strongly associated with patterns of consumption of animal fats in the distant past (1965), but not with consumption of animal fats in the more recent past (1988). Concentrations of blood cholesterol were available from 13 of the countries. Again, death rates in 1992 were strongly associated with cholesterol concentrations in 1970, but not with cholesterol concentrations in 1990. The time lag was thus about 25 years. It evidently takes time for animal fats to kill you, quick as death might be when it does come. Other English epidemiologists arrived at similar conclusions from analyses of the relationship of smoking to cancer of the lung. They found that current risk of lung cancer is determined by the smoking habits 30–40 years earlier.[16] When so many years elapse between transgression and retribution, it is not surprising that so many of us have been in doubt about the connection.

Have patterns of food consumption in populations changed in a manner compatible with a rise in coronary artery disease beginning in the first decades of the twentieth century in the United States and in the economically developed countries of Europe? Systematic estimates of what whole populations have eaten at any one time were not done until the late 19th century. An estimate of this sort was provided in 1881 by a

Committee of the British Association.[17] It was later revised to allow comparisons with later estimates. Between 1880 and the period 1909–1928, annual consumption of meat per Englishman increased from 40 to 59 kg. Consumption of sugar also increased substantially, and consumption of potatoes decreased substantially, whereas the increases in consumption of milk and butter were slower and did not reach maximum until 1950. Overall, therefore, the food patterns really did seem to have changed in a manner consistent with the proposition that an increase in the consumption of animal fats late in the 19th century, consequent to industrialization and increasing affluence, caused coronary artery disease 25 years later. All of this must have happened gradually. The Committee of the British Association believed that their 1880 estimates already showed that Englishmen were eating more: "*A large consumption of articles of food in great part imported is a sign of general prosperity, and is conclusive (sic!) to greater effectiveness of labour. There is no reason to suppose that home production has diminished of late years, except indeed as the consequence of deficient harvests on special years. The increasing imports therefore denote so much additional food consumed by the people*".

The fall in the incidence of coronary artery disease in the last decades of the 20th century could also, at least in part, be due to changes in diet. Ascertaining such changes in national diet continues to be extremely difficult, however. Although the United States Department of Agriculture provides measures of per capita availability of several hundred different foods, as an example, it is uncertain how much of the different foods is actually eaten. According to a recent analysis from the University of Minnesota in Minneapolis, from the period 1970–1974 to 1995 there were distinct falls in the average per capita availability of several foods known to promote coronary artery disease. As examples, the availability of red meat fell from 59 to 52 kg and whole milk from 90 to 33 kg per capita, and the percentage of total energy from fat also decreased. The data also suggested that intakes of saturated fatty acids had declined, while intakes of monounsaturated and polyunsaturated fat had increased.[18] The latter finding probably reflects an increase in the use of vegetable oils, at the expense of animal fat, that had begun much earlier in the century.[19] All in all, these data, uncertain as they are, are consistent with declining concentrations of blood cholesterol[20] and declining rates of coronary artery disease in the United States and elsewhere in the developed world during the last decades of the 20th century.

The astute reader will remark here that time lag seems to apply to the increase in coronary artery disease but not to the decrease in the disease. Trials of lowering cholesterol with drugs and diet show that the disease in the coronary arteries can be stopped and sometimes even reversed within a year or two. Law and Wald therefore remark that "*slow inception and rapid reversal are not inconsistent, and one should not be used to suggest that the other is incorrect. The relative risk of smoking related diseases also increases slowly after starting smoking but falls soon after stopping smoking*".

We'll discuss the trials of cholesterol lowering in a later chapter. In the remainder of this one, however, let us question why coronary artery disease appears slowly but can be made to disappear quickly. Once again, the answer is in the pathology.

Pathology

We already noted some of the essential features of atherosclerosis in the previous chapter. Imagine that you are a pathologist doing a routine postmortem examination of an old person. You have opened the heart, and you have seen that the chambers are fairly normal. Now you insert the point of one of the blades of the scissors into a coronary artery, and you open the artery longitudinally. All of it is more or less atherosclerotic. In some places the wall of the artery is almost normal, but in others it is markedly thickened, and here and there the wall is hard and crunchy because of calcification. Wherever the atherosclorosis is most advanced, we speak of atheromas or athero-sclerotic plaques. An atheroma is an abnormal growth in the wall of the artery. Inside the atheroma is a little pocket of material with the consistency of toothpaste. It is composed of cholesterol and dead cells. It does little harm if it is encapsulated by hard fibrous tissue so that it is not in contact with the blood flowing through the artery. If the hard tissue becomes inflamed, however, the capsule can weaken and rupture, allowing the "toothpaste" to come into contact with the blood. When that happens, blood rapidly forms a clot, which is also called a thrombus. Sometimes the clot just further narrows the artery, but at other times it closes the artery off completely.

Some of this was apparent to scientists of the 19th century. Rudolf Virchov in Berlin described thrombosis in terms of damage to the vessel wall, components of blood and the flow of blood through the blood vessel. He had convinced physicians that most diseases had a cellular basis, and in the case of thrombotic disease he showed that clotting of blood involved not only the white cells of blood but also tiny fragments of cells called platelets. When the wall of an artery or a vein is somehow damaged, white cells and platelets quickly attach to the damaged part. The platelets stick together, and they form a clot with a variety of blood proteins called coagulation factors. The purpose of the clot is to stop bleeding from a damaged blood vessel, a process without which an animal would die shortly after birth.

Clotting can also happen if an artery has been damaged by disease such as atherosclerosis, however. In that case, clotting can be what closes the artery and kills the animal. In this and so many other areas of medicine, one man's remedy is another man's poison. Physiological mechanisms, which increased the chances of survival during the long periods of formation of the genome, become part and parcel of disease in a modern world of affluence, physical inactivity and longevity that is very different from the world of the hunter-gatherer. It is, fundamentally, for this reason that drugs to combat thrombosis, especially the coumadins, must be dosed so carefully as to inhibit clotting without causing bleeding. In an earlier age of decadence, the Romans knew that anything can be poisonous, depending on the dose administered ("*dosis sola facit venena*").[21]

By the end of the 20th century, thrombosis and inflammation were understood in rich detail, even though satisfactory medical control of both processes remained elusive. Thrombosis and inflammation have turned out to be important for many reasons. One reason is that understanding inflammation and thrombosis opens new avenues for pharmacological treatment of atherosclerosis. Another reason, and the one pertinent to the present discussion, is that inflammation and thrombosis explain the rapid phase of atherosclerotic disease: rupture of an inflamed capsule precipitates clotting. It takes only seconds to minutes for a small clot to form. It is therefore quite possible that only part of the disease process has undergone most of the apparent change during the 20th century. That part could be the pocket of *"toothpaste"*, inflammation with capsule rupture, and thrombosis. Another part, the gradual thickening of the wall of the artery by stable fibrous tissue, could have developed pretty well as it may have done before the epidemic of coronary artery disease.

There is only one study of the frequency of coronary atherosclerosis over long periods of time. It is an older study and less than perfect by contemporary methodological standards, but the results can be understood in terms of the dichotomy between the slow and rapid phases of atherosclerosis and thrombosis. Let us go back to the first half of the 20th century. That is when most of the rise of coronary artery disease occurred.

Jeremy N. Morris studied 1,405 post-mortem reports of London Hospital in the six year periods 1908–1913 and 1944–1949.[22] There were 995 reports from the early period and 410 reports from the later period. Morris was surprised when he saw that, in persons dead for whatever reason, there had been a decline in the prevalence of severe coronary atherosclerosis during that 36 year period. That result certainly did not tally very well with the perception that the disease was on the increase. The result was different, however, when he counted the patients in whom the post-mortem examination showed that they in fact had died of coronary artery disease (recent coronary thrombosis or acute myocardial infarction). The number of such patients had increased in the same hospital in the same period. Morris therefore believed that the incidence of stable coronary artery disease had not increased in the forty years up to 1949. The part of the disease that had increased was thrombosis and myocardial infarction. That viewpoint did not gather much of a following at the time, but it is quite reasonable in the light of more recent research into atherosclerosis. *"Certainly the disease did not suddenly leap into existence about 1920, fully armed for destruction like Athena from the brow of Zeus".*[23]

As late as 1990, we had expected that if reversal of atherosclerotic disease was possible at all, it might well take as long as it had taken for the disease to develop in the first place, decades rather than years. Research of the last decade of the century changed that view completely, so that the overall picture is now consistent with the rapid fluctuations in disease rates seen in some countries right after World War II and with the data from London Hospital.

The first experimental data to support the idea of a rapidly changing and a slowly changing component of the disease were from arteriographic studies. "Arteriography" literally means depiction of an artery. In this case, the coronary arteries are depicted by injecting a small amount of fluid, opaque to x-rays, into the coronary arteries so that the cavity of the artery turns up white on an x-ray film. In a typical study of this sort, researchers performed coronary arteriographies before and after two years of treatment of heart patients with a cholesterol-lowering drug or an inactive control tablet (placebo). In almost all of the studies, treatment widened the white lines on the x-ray films that represented the cavities of the coronary arteries, but the improvements were very small indeed. That was disappointing, and the researchers were therefore pleasantly surprised to see that there were fewer heart attacks and deaths in the group of patients that had been treated with active drug. This makes sense, however, if the arteriographic appearances reflect the slow, stable and mostly innocuous component of atherosclerosis, and the reduction in rates of heart attacks and deaths reflects the fast component of atheroma, inflammation and thrombosis.

Although these arteriographic studies had involved about 6,000 patients in all, they were still considered too small to establish to everyone's satisfaction that coronary artery disease could be prevented or reversed by lowering cholesterol. Simultaneously, however, much larger clinical trials had been started. They did not necessarily involve arteriographies, but they were of longer duration, and ultimately they involved more than 50,000 patients. By 2002, six trials of this sort had shown that cholesterol-lowering treatment really did lower rates of heart attacks and deaths.[24,25]

Again, it was remarkable how quickly that took place. Although each trial lasted about five years, the duration of exposure to active or control treatment in those patients who died or had a heart attack had been only half the trial length. This subtle point, made by Malcom Law, is almost always missed, but it is obvious when you think about it. It is evident that a death means that a patient can no longer be in the trial, but the same applies to a heart attack, even if it does not kill the patient. In technical terms, deaths and heart attacks are both trial "end-points". The point made by Malcom Law is that the first heart attack or death might occur the day after the trial is begun, and that event must be entered into the trial data base, even though it is unlikely that exposure to either placebo or active drug could have made any difference after only one day. The last heart attack or death might occur the day before the trial ends, and that "end-point" must of course also be entered into the trial data base. In patients suffering end-point events, therefore, the average duration of exposure to treatment with either placebo or active treatment is only one half of the length of the trial. Most of the cholesterol-lowering trials lasted about five years, and patients who died or suffered heart attacks had therefore been exposed to placebo or active drug for an average period of only $2\frac{1}{2}$ years.

If one looks more closely at what is going on in the arteries, two major findings of the last two decades of research help to explain why atherosclerotic disease is so much more amenable to treatment than we had imagined not so long ago. The first is that the innermost layer of the arteries, the endothelial layer, has turned out to be a very dynamic part of the artery wall. It is composed of just one layer of cells, the endothelial cells, so it is extremely thin. Whereas cells in organs like the thyroid gland secrete hormones that travel through the blood stream to other organs, the endothelial cells secrete hormones that travel only fractions of a millimeter into the artery wall to cause it to dilate or constrict, permitting more or less blood to flow through the artery. That control deteriorates during the very early stages of atherosclerosis, but it has now turned out that it can be reestablished in the course of weeks by drugs that lower cholesterol.

The second is the inflammatory aspect of atherosclerosis. I have alluded to it several times, and I should now provide a bit of explanation. Cholesterol and other lipids (fats) are transported in the blood attached to different proteins. The resulting complex of molecules of lipids and proteins is called a lipoprotein. A few lipoproteins continuously enter into the artery wall from the blood, and most of them also leave the artery wall again. A very small proportion of them is retained in the inner layers of the artery wall, however, because they are caught by certain sugary proteins (glycoproteins) in the fluid separating the cells of the wall. It is especially lipoproteins of low density (low density lipoproteins, or LDL) that are liable to get caught in this way.

Unable to get back into the blood stream, LDL initiate a series of events in the artery wall that ultimately result in formation of an atherosclerotic plaque. Chemical modification of the structure of LDL by oxidation, attachment of sugars, or enzymatic degradation appear to enhance the ability of LDL to cause atherosclerosis. Such chemically modified lipoproteins attract specialized muscle cells called "smooth muscle cells" from other layers of the artery wall, where they normally do the work of dilating or constricting the artery to honor the needs of the various parts of the body for more or less blood. From the blood the modified lipoproteins also attract white cells, whose normal function it is to seek out and destroy foreign substances. The smooth muscle cells form the sclerotic, or hard, part of atherosclerosis. The white cells gorge themselves on the modified LDL, so that they turn into huge, fat-filled cells. They are called foam cells because, under the microscope, they look as if they had been filled with white foam. When they have become fully satiated with LDL, the foam cells burst and release their contents of cholesterol and other fats into the fluid between the cells. The soft, toothpaste-like core of the atheroma is composed of this debris of cholesterol, other fats and dead foam cells.

The presence of white cells identifies the whole process as an inflammatory one. The white cells produce an array of biochemical substances called cytokines, some of which are able to break down parts of the artery wall. That is what weakens the capsule so that it can rupture and expose the toothpaste-like core of the atheroma to the blood rushing through the cavity of the artery. The various kinds of white cells collaborate with each other to do this, but first they must be activated by an antigen, a protein that the cells perceive as foreign and something to destroy. A literally burning question is which antigens activate the white cells to begin the inflammatory process. An obvious candidate is the LDL. The white cells probably perceive it as foreign, because it has been chemically modified, for example by oxidation or by attachment of a sugar molecule. There are other candidates, however. They include proteins that normally reside inside cells but are released when cells die, and they include various infectious agents.

At least three viruses (Marek's disease virus, herpes virus and cytomegalovirus) and two microbes (Chlamydia and Helicobacter) are candidates as activators of white cells, and small trials of antibiotic treatment to kill the microbes have suggested that such treatment might help patients with coronary heart disease. Larger trials are underway to confirm or refute that idea. If confirmed, an infectious agent might be invoked to explain the rise and fall of coronary heart disease in the 20th century, but at the time of writing, the infection theory of atherosclerosis is not well supported by experimental data.

Since many different antigens might be able to activate white cells in atherosclerosis, the hunt for just one culpable antigen might ultimately prove to be in vain.[26] At present, however, the most likely candidate for the role as chief arsonist is chemically modified LDL. Depending on the balance of these many components and processes, athero-sclerotic plaques vary greatly in their composition, architecture and structural stability. They tend to be stable if they have sparse lipid atheroma but heavy fibrous tissue with many smooth muscle cells and few white cells. Such stable plaques can narrow the artery and cause angina pectoris. They rarely occlude the artery, however, and they are not prone to rupture. In contrast, atheromas with a high content of lipids and white cells are unstable, and they easily precipitate closure of an artery to the heart muscle, to the brain or to another organ. The result is an infarct of the heart, of the brain or of another organ. If the occlusion is not complete, it can produce short but frightening bouts of angina pectoris or blindness or paralysis. They are due to repeated cycles of formation and spontaneous dissolution of the clot, and they require quick treatment to avert a definitive myocardial infarct or stroke.

The age-adjusted data from the epidemiological, clinical and basic research of the last decade of the 20th century are compatible with the idea that atherosclerosis can rapidly be rendered much less dangerous. As depicted by arteriography, it does not disappear, but it stabilizes: rupture of plaques and ensuing thrombosis occur much less frequently. This is not only good news for patients with atherosclerosis of the coronary and other arteries. It also explains why the clinical manifestations of the disease could increase and later decrease so dramatically in the developed countries of the 20th century, despite an almost unchanged degree of stable coronary artery disease as demonstrated in mid-century by the London Hospital study and in the last decade of the last century by the arteriographic studies.

These and countless other insights into the causes of atherosclerosis are real scientific advances. They would suggest that coronary artery disease as a clinical entity now should be definitively on the retreat as it has been in the developed countries during the last 30 years of the 20th century.

Why the Decline of Coronary Artery Disease Might Have Stopped

Coronary artery disease may no longer be on the retreat, however. A new scenario for coronary artery disease emerged at the close of the 20th century. Data, in particular from the United States, suggest that the continued fall in age-adjusted rates of deaths due to coronary artery disease has stopped.[27] There are several reasons for the renewed strength of the disease, some bad, some good.

One reason of major concern is that the smoking of tobacco, although declining in the developed world, is on the increase in the developing world. Another is that we are getting fatter, and in Europe and the United States, increasingly widespread obesity and diabetes are almost certain to herald a come-back for coronary artery disease. This pattern will probably be repeated all over the world, because obesity and diabetes are on the increase as affluence comes to China, India and some of the other developing countries. How dangerous it is to be obese depends on how the fat is distributed in your body. It is especially dangerous if a lot of it is lodged between the organs in your abdomen, a common cause of the pouch of middle-aged men. Not only does belly fat raise blood pressure, blood glucose and blood lipids, it also causes the liver to produce substances that inflame the artery wall. Caesar felt most comfortable with fat, cheerful people around him. So might we, but some of that cheery inner warmth might shorten life.

Not all is so threatening, however. We are getting better at detecting the disease, and we are getting better at treating it. As we have already seen, both advances cause the disease to become more common, but let us elaborate a little on that apparently paradoxical phenomenon.

A disease appears to be more common if we adopt new and wider definitions for detecting it, and, indeed, the criteria for diagnosing coronary heart disease have changed very recently. The measurements of transaminases, discussed earlier in this chapter, have been replaced by more sensitive measurements of proteins called troponins. Like transaminases, troponins are released from the cells of heart muscle when they die. The sensitivity of troponin measurements is so great that death of less than 1% of heart muscle can now be detected easily. This means that an attack of chest pain, which in 1980 could have been dismissed as innocuous and unexplained, now qualifies as a heart attack (a myocardial infarction). More people will therefore be identified as heart patients, because they have survived a heart attack.[28]

Our ability to diagnose coronary artery disease is also improving. It is now possible to detect atherosclerosis of the coronary arteries by sophisticated x-ray machines, nuclear magnetic resonance scanners and other instruments long before the appearance of symptoms of coronary heart disease. I alluded to these improvements in diagnostic instruments in the introduction to this book. Emphasis will therefore increasingly be on the detection, not only of coronary *heart* disease, but also of coronary *artery* disease, and more people will therefore be identified as having coronary disease. Calcification of the coronary arteries, which can be detected easily by x-ray machines (CT scanners), is a rough measure of coronary artery disease. It is probably about five times more common than coronary heart disease.[29]

Treatment has also improved. Patients survive the first heart attack more often now than they did 30 to 50 years ago. By definition, however, they survive as patients with coronary disease, and thus they also enlarge the proportion of the population with the disease. To be sure, they may be distressed by angina pectoris and symptoms of heart failure, and they might require surgical and medical treatment, but they are alive. People are living longer for many other reasons, moreover, and since atherosclerosis becomes increasingly common with advancing age, coronary artery disease will for that reason also affect an increasing proportion of the population.

It would be nice to know whether the apparent prolongation of the epidemic of coronary artery disease in the developed countries is mainly due to obesity and smoking or whether it is mainly due to better diagnosis and better survival. We shall therefore close this chapter as it began, with some uncertainty about whether the continuation of the epidemic of coronary artery disease is more apparent than real. We now have excellent methods, CT scanning especially, with which to resolve some of this uncertainty in sufficiently large, well-designed and carefully executed prospective epidemiological studies. It is not easy, though, to obtain funding for this kind of research. Less sexy and commercially less interesting than molecular biology, basic epidemiology is nevertheless more important if we are convinced that coronary artery disease is a serious public health issue.

Chapter 3

Coronary Artery Disease After 2000: Epidemiologic Transitions

In the first two chapters we traced the history of coronary artery disease from about 1500 B.C. until the present. The disease was certainly with us before that history began, however, and it is certain to be with us in the future. The question is how prevalent it will be. The World Health Organization of the United Nations predicts that the disease will continue its advance across the planet during the first two decades of the 21st century. By 2020 it is expected to top the list of diseases burdening the health systems of the world.

A development of this magnitude must interest those entrusted with the planning of health care systems, and it clear that the major professional societies of cardiology[1] and the pharmaceutical industry already have plans in place to adjust themselves to the world-wide epidemic of coronary artery disease. In the Summer of 2002, the Council of the European Union approved a "Heart Plan for Europe" that had been developed by the European Society of Cardiology. To combat "today's Black Death", the plan calls for a reduction of blood cholesterol in individuals to 5.0 mmol/l by 2007, for a reduction of blood pressure to less than 140/90 mm Hg in individuals younger than 65 years of age, and for a reduction in the number of cigarette smokers in Europe by 1% each year.[2]

Given the scope, not only of the WHO predictions themselves, but also of the political conclusions now being drawn from them, it is important to understand how they were made. The WHO prediction concerning coronary heart disease was only one of the results of a large study of the global patterns of disease likely to occur between 1990 and 2020. The study was performed by epidemiologists at the Harvard School of Public Health and the WHO, and the World Bank was a third partner. Called the Global Burden of Disease Study, it has been published in book form[3] and in a series of summary articles in the Lancet. It was performed by Christopher J. L. Murray and Allan D. Lopez, who divided the world into 8 major regions:

(1) the established market economies of Western Europe and North America;
(2) the former socialist economies of Eastern Europe;
(3) Latin America and the Caribbean;
(4) China;
(5) India;
(6) the middle eastern crescent (North Africa, the Middle East, Pakistan, Central Asian Republics);

(7) the rest of Asia and the Pacific islands; and

(8) sub-Saharan Africa.

Diseases were divided into three broad categories: communicable (infectious) diseases, non-communicable diseases such as cardiovascular disease and cancer, and intentional and non-intentional injuries. The data were the best available from national and regional death registries. Some regions of the world had virtually no reliable mortality or morbidity data, and it was therefore necessary to make several assumptions.

The study was based on a computer model of how changes in the occurrence of many different diseases will affect millions of people in the different regions of the world over a long period of time. One of the important concepts in the study was the idea of "epidemiologic transitions," which is also at the core of policies currently being developed by the WHO. Epidemiologic disease transitions are said to occur when historical changes in our environment cause one dominant class of diseases to be succeeded by another. For example, increasing affluence has improved housing, clothing, food supply and medicines so that infectious disease could be combated more effectively. At the same time, however, by supplying food in abundance and by eliminating the need for manual labor, affluence has increased life expectancy and set the scene for degenerative diseases such as coronary heart disease and cancer. Indeed, the major current transition affecting the developed and developing countries is from a period dominated by infectious diseases to one dominated by degenerative diseases.

Like other transitions in human history, it is not happening at the same time in all human populations. In the established market economies of the developed countries such as North America and Western Europe, it happened in the first half of the 20th century, but in the developing economies of Africa, it is just beginning to happen at the beginning of the 21st century. Within cardiovascular medicine itself, the transition is exemplified by the succession of rheumatic heart disease by coronary heart disease. Epidemiologists have thought in terms of four stages of diseases, and more recently, Salim Yusuf at McMaster University in Hamilton, Ontario in Canada and Srinath Reddy of the All India Institute of Medical Sciences in New Delhi have proposed that a fifth should be added to the list.[4,5]

Infectious diseases and nutritional deficiencies dominate the first stage. Large parts of Sub-Sahara as well as rural areas of South America and Asia are still in this stage, whereas China and other Asian countries have advanced to the second stage. In terms of cardiovascular disease, the second stage is characterized by diseases related to hypertension. An example is stroke due to bleeding into the brain. As life expectancy continues to improve, there is the transition to the third stage, which is dominated by cancer and atherosclerotic diseases due to smoking, physical inactivity and fatty foods. Urban India, Latin America and the former socialist countries have arrived at this stage, which is followed by a fourth stage presently being enjoyed by Western Europe, North America, Australia and New Zealand. At this fourth stage, preventive and therapeutic medicine is able to delay most of the signs and symptoms of cardiovascular diseases until old age. The fifth stage proposed by Yusuf and Reddy is a resurgence, due to social upheaval and war, of conditions seen in the first two stages. They believe that Russia at the turn of the century could represent this stage.

Death is not the only relevant measure of disease severity. Disease also disables, and severe disability of long duration can burden health care systems more than a quick death. One can imagine, however, that perception of severity of disability could vary a lot between peoples of different cultures. That turned out not to be the case in the Global Burden of Disease Study. The researchers asked health care professionals from different countries to grade different kinds of disability, and it was apparent that estimates of degree and duration of disability due to different diseases did not differ very much between countries. To take an extreme example, irrespective of the cultural setting, the consequences of a stroke were considered to be more serious than vitiligo, a loss of skin pigment.

All of the data were then modeled by computer, based partly on a large number of parameters and assumptions, and partly on a procedure to ensure that there was internal consistency between all the calculations. It would exceed the limits of this chapter to attempt to describe the projections made by the Global Burden of Disease Study. In the context of this discussion, the important part of the study's vision of the future is, that communicable diseases are likely to continue to decline to be replaced by non-communicable diseases and violence as causes of death and disability. These two measures of suffering are incorporated in the concept of "disability-adjusted-life-years". That term, taken straight out of health economic jargon, denotes the sum of years of life lost and years of life lived with disability.

The Global Burden of Disease Study predicts that, between 1990 and 2020, this world-wide sum of disability-adjusted-life-years will be largely unchanged, increasing only from 1.38 to 1.39 billion. Within that sum, however, the percentage of disability-adjusted-life-years due to communicable disease will decrease from 43.9% to 20.1%, that due to non-communicable disease will increase from 40.9% to 59.7% and that due to violence will increase from 15.2% to 20.1%. Coronary artery disease will maintain its position as the single most important cause of death, but it will advance from fourth to first in the ranking of disease by disability-adjusted-life-years. The authors of the study ascribe this to the widening epidemic of tobacco smoking and the ageing of all populations of the world.

They offer three alternative projections, differing mainly in the degree of optimism regarding the prospects for a continuing decline in infectious diseases, and they emphasize that several features of the study introduce particular uncertainties. They are the epidemic of AIDS, the rates of intentional injury, and the relationships of infectious to other diseases. An example of the latter relationship is hepatitis B, an infectious disease in its own right, but also a cause of another disease, namely cancer of the liver. Although not an infectious disease, diabetes also exemplifies a disease in its own right which simultaneously causes another disease, namely coronary artery disease. Finally, uncertainties were introduced by the choices of assumptions and mathematical models. The projections are therefore "three visions of the future — the numerical consequences of the set of assumptions and methods used to generate these visions".

The Global Burden of Disease Study is a self-contained model of global disease development. By far the most comprehensive model currently available, it can be modified as we learn more about the causes and possibilities of prevention or treatment of any one disease. For our present purposes, however, it is important to note that the explanations given for the expectation of a continued epidemic of coronary heart disease are implicit in the model, because the effects of tobacco and the results of ageing of populations were already factored into it.

Not factored into the model is the potential for pharmacological treatment and widespread dietary change. Since drugs and food both can affect the rapidly changing part of the atherosclerotic process, reviewed in the preceding chapters, whatever happens in medicine and agriculture could result in changes in disease rates of a magnitude similar to those that we have seen in the 20th century.

The idea that some sort of medical intervention can solve a major public health problem is not equally acceptable everywhere. In Europe, many people recoil from it, but it seems to be more acceptable in the United States, and the World Health Organization has a commendably pragmatic view of cost-effective drug therapies as a part of comprehensive policies to promote health across the globe.[6] In some of the following chapters I shall discuss the statin trials as examples of major advances in pharmacological research. Shortly after the first of them had shown that the course of coronary artery disease could be arrested and even reversed, the American Nobel laureates, Michael Brown and Joseph Goldstein, suggested that the disease might be gone with the 20th century.[7] The suggestion was provocative but not facetious. The statin drugs seem to be quite safe, and, inadvisably in my view, they might soon become available at low cost over the counter. If available to a sufficiently large proportion of most populations, they could check the disease on a large scale in both the developed and the developing countries.

Widespread dietary change could also affect the progress of coronary artery disease across the planet. The World Health Organization and the Food and Agricultural Organization are both parts of the United Nations, and they have published their views of what is likely to happen to patterns of human disease[3] and to patterns of food consumption by humans[8] in the first decades of the 21st century. In a later chapter we shall discuss the projected huge increase in production of livestock across the planet, especially in the Far East. That development alone will contribute importantly to the anticipated spread of coronary artery disease, but it has not been factored into either the WHO projections or, to my knowledge, the plans of any public health authority.

More dramatic developments in agriculture are also possible. There will be widespread famine, for example, if industrialized agriculture breaks down. In that case, coronary artery disease will be the least of our problems. Calamities of this sort form no part of the projections of developments made by institutions like the WHO and the Food and Agricultural Organization, because the projections are orderly extrapolations of trends that are already apparent.

Impressive progress is probable, and calamities are certain, but both are unpredictable as to where, when and to whom. In 1900, readers of Jules Verne and H. G. Wells could anticipate some of the spectacular progress of the science and technology of the 20th century, but there was no Cassandra to say that the European order including four empires would collapse within 20 years. Nor did many anticipate, at the beginning of 2000, that President Mugabe would intentionally dismantle Zimbabwean agriculture two years later.

Chapter 4

The Cholesterol Controversy

Patients would be right to lodge complaints if physicians and nurses in surgical and obstetric wards failed to wash their hands before examinations or operations. And in cardiology departments, patients are right to expect physicians and nurses to tell them how they are most likely to avoid another myocardial infarction: don't smoke, keep up the good work on diet, don't forget the betablocker to keep heart rhythm normal and the statin to lower cholesterol. And much more. Come back in three weeks.

Yet there was once bitter controversy about the utility of antisepsis, the merits of lowering cholesterol, and the value of countless other principles of modern medicine that now are taken for granted. It is not difficult to see why. While the agents of some diseases are evident — violence as a cause of injury for example — the agents of other diseases are invisible. For sure, cholesterol can be measured by chemical assay, and bacteria can be studied under a microscope, but neither cholesterol nor bacteria are part of direct human experience.

Before anything about bacteria was really known, childbed fever was thought to be due to "miasma", which means noxious atmosphere. It was a fuzzy idea invoked to explain several different diseases that could not be understood before the advent of microbiology. Malaria literally means bad air. Chiefs of obstetric clinics believed in the miasma theory of childbed fever, and they resigned themselves to the appallingly high rates of deaths of mothers soon after delivery. When Ignaz Semmelweis showed them how to avoid childbed fever in 1848, they did not believe him.

The controversy surrounding antisepsis in the 19th century and the fate of Ignaz Semmelweis are classics of medicine, and they can be understood within the context of the state of science and perhaps also the state of politics in which they occurred. In the 1840s, most women in Vienna had their babies delivered at home, but some were forced by poverty or illegitimacy to go into hospital. In hospital one in five died of childbed fever. Semmelweis worked in such a hospital. He observed that childbed fever was 2 to 3 times more common in the ward where the medical students received their training than in the ward where midwives received their training. It occurred to him that the students might be transmitting a noxious and fatal agent to the women in the delivery room from the autopsy rooms where they dissected corpses including the bodies of women who had recently died of childbed fever. When he directed the students to wash their hands in chlorinated water before the examination of women in labor, death rates immediately fell from 18% to 1%.

That was in 1848, the year of political rebellion throughout Europe. Semmelweis had participated in the rebellions in Vienna, and when he spoke and wrote about his work on antisepsis, the medical faculty in Vienna, opposed to his political ideas, also rejected his medical and scientific ideas, and when he was offered a senior position it was only on humiliating terms. He retired to his native city of Pest in Hungary, the subservient partner in the Austro-Hungarian empire. As professor of obstetrics in Pest, he continued to argue for antisepsis, but as late as 1857 the editor of the Wiener Medizinische Wochenschrift wrote that it was time to stop the nonsense about the chlorine hand wash. The controversy wore him down, he suffered a mental breakdown, and in 1865 Semmelweis died in a psychiatric hospital.

Physicians ultimately accepted the principles of antisepsis, in part because of the work of Joseph Lister in Great Britain, in part also because of the emergence of the methods of modern bacteriology such as the cultivation of bacteria on plates of nutrient gelatin and stains to visualize them for microscopy. That was in the 1870s. Thirty years earlier, Semmelweis had not only lacked acceptable political and perhaps ethnic credentials, he had also worked in a discipline without the methods and the concepts with which to explain his findings.

The controversy surrounding cholesterol in the 20th century was more complicated, it lasted much longer, and the changes in death rates brought about by the lowering of cholesterol in blood plasma were not nearly as dramatic as those brought about by antisepsis. However, the cholesterol controversy was also propagated and in part also ultimately resolved by forces extraneous to the science. By 1975, the evidence was more than sufficient to persuade thoughtful people that cholesterol in blood plasma (plasma cholesterol or "blood cholesterol") should be lowered to prevent coronary artery disease, but it took years of more research to convince physicians that cholesterol is one of the causes of the disease and that lowering cholesterol can prevent it. To appreciate how remarkably late the controversy was resolved, let us briefly summarize the evidence and then consider the reasons why it took so much effort and so much time for physicians to accept it.

The evidence connecting cholesterol to atherosclerosis emerged from many different kinds of research. It required numerous studies of lowering cholesterol by diet or drugs, studies of human populations, of patients with a rare genetic disease, of corpses and of many different laboratory animals. To use a favorite cliché of scientific writing, it required numerous lines of evidence. They all had to be brought together into one overall concept.

Man's Experiments With Animals

The story ended where most science is now done, in the medico-industrial complex, but it began by chance in a military setting in the first decade of the 20th century. In the Department of Internal Medicine of the Military Academy Saint Petersburg in Russia, a young clinical assistant, Dr. Ignatowsky, was interested in kidney disease. He was particularly interested in the effects that food with a lot of protein might have on metabolism and on kidney function. He therefore fed meat, milk and eggs to rabbits and observed what happened. The most striking thing he saw was not kidney disease, however. Instead it was atherosclerosis of the aorta. The disease in the rabbits resembled atherosclerosis in humans, and Ignatowsky thought that it was due to the proteins that he had fed to the animals. A few years later, however, a colleague working in the Institute of Experimental Medicine in Saint Petersburg, Nikolai N. Anitschkov, definitively shifted the focus of research from protein to cholesterol when he showed that the atherosclerosis could be produced in the rabbits simply by feeding them pure cholesterol.[1]

Since then, observations and experiments in birds, rodents and non-human primates have confirmed the relationship of high blood cholesterol to atherosclerosis. Chicken, quail and pigeons have a naturally occurring high cholesterol in blood plasma, and several breeds of these species of birds develop atherosclerosis spontaneously. It develops faster if they are fed cholesterol, however, and feeding laboratory animals cholesterol and saturated fat is a standard method by which to produce experimental atherosclerosis. In fact, there is no atherosclerosis to study in laboratory animals unless their cholesterol levels have been made to rise in some way. That has been known since the work of Anitschkow at the time of the outbreak of World War I.

Researchers must still increase the concentrations of blood cholesterol in order to study atherosclerosis. This is the age of molecular biology, however, and the way cholesterol is made to rise nowadays is far more sophisticated than Anitschkow could have imagined. It is done, not only by feeding and by classical breeding techniques, but also by genetic engineering of the genes that code for proteins and enzymes involved in the metabolism of cholesterol.

Humans have employed breeding for about 10,000 years in order to create animals and plants that are very different from their wild ancestors. For example, corn and wheat are very different from wild ancestor grasses, and anyone who has seen a Mexican Chihuahua will know how far breeding can bring dogs from ancestral wild dogs like the wolf. The breeding of animals employs controlled mating followed by a selection of offspring for further mating. By breeding, traits considered desirable by the breeder can emerge over the course of several generations.

The results can be very impressive when the methods of genetic engineering are added to those of breeding. Leaving aside the enormous differences in methods, the results of breeding only and those of genetic engineering plus breeding can differ in two important respects. First, breeding usually results in gradations of differences between ancestor and progeny, because they are due to small effects of changes in many different genes rather than to a major effect of a change in one gene. Secondly, genetic engineering plus breeding can introduce genes into animals from completely different species of animals. For example, human genes can be introduced into experimental animals by genetic engineering. The resulting "transgenic" animals can define the role of the gene in question, and they could not have been created by breeding only.

Transgenic animals are created by injecting the gene of interest (the transgene) into a fertilized egg cell, which is then placed in the oviduct of a female animal. Of the animals born and weaned, about 30% will have the transgene somewhere in their genome, and the transgene will be passed on to their offspring. The methodology is demanding and requires large research operations. Even more demanding are gene knock-out experiments, which until recently could be carried out only in mice. A gene can be "knocked out" by a piece of specialised DNA inserted into embryonic stem cells, which can develop into cells of the different organs of a whole animal. If the gene of the animal's germ cells (sperm cells and egg cells) has been knocked out, mating will produce offspring lacking the gene in all organs.

Even on a normal diet of mouse chow, concentrations of blood cholesterol are high in mice without the gene for apolipoprotein E, which is one of the proteins that binds to the LDL receptor, mentioned briefly in Chapter 2. Cholesterol soars to very high levels, however, when such apoE knock-out mice are fed chow resembling the typical diet consumed by Danish and American humans. The mice then develop severe atherosclerosis which in most respects is quite similar to that in humans. Such animals have been used, for example, to study the possible role of microbes like Chlamydia in atherosclerosis, but the important thing to keep in mind is that high levels of blood cholesterol, obtained by diet or genetic manipulation or both, have been a necessary condition for these studies. There would have been no atherosclerosis to study if the blood cholesterol had not been increased by breeding, by genetic manipulation or by feeding the animals chow resembling the food that we eat.

Thus, a fundamental element of modern research into atherosclerosis, raising the level of cholesterol in the blood of the experimental animal, is the same as it was nearly a hundred years ago. As a trade secret of the experimentalist, however, that insight has had no great impact on clinical medicine or public health policy.

Nature's Experiments With Man

Humans experiment with animals, and nature has experimented with us. Familial hypercholesterolemia is the most common of the experiments of nature demonstrating how cholesterol and other components of lipoproteins cause atherosclerosis in humans. The term denotes the familial occurrence of high concentrations of blood cholesterol. It is usually caused by a mutation in the gene that codes for the LDL receptor, which is a protein in the membrane surrounding cells. Liver cells use it to pick up LDL from blood. If the gene that tells the cell how to make the LDL receptor is abnormal, there may be no LDL receptors at all, or they may in some way be unable to perform their normal task of removing LDL from the fluid surrounding the cells. Concentrations of LDL in blood are then also high. Approximately one in 500 people in most populations have inherited an abnormal gene for the LDL receptor from one of their parents. They are said to have the heterozygous form of the disease. In an environment of food plenty it causes early atherosclerosis and death by coronary disease in middle adulthood at rates up to 100 times of those in people with normal blood cholesterol. The rare patients with homozygous familial hypercholesterolemia (approximately one in a million people) have inherited abnormal genes from both parents. Concentrations of LDL in the blood are then extremely high, and if the patients are not treated, few of them survive their 30th birthday. Some die of coronary artery diseases in childhood.

Siegfried Josef Thannhauser, working in the United States, and Carl Müller in Oslo, Norway, had characterized the disease in clinical and elementary biochemical terms before World War II,[2,3] but it was not until 1973 that it was understood on the molecular level. In the autumn of that year, Joseph Goldstein and Michael Brown of Texas

University in Dallas reported the discovery of the LDL receptor, which heralded the age of molecular medicine, and for which Goldstein and Brown were awarded the Nobel Prize in Medicine in 1986.[4] Familial hypercholesterolemia should long ago have sufficed to convince physicians that high blood cholesterol in humans causes atherosclerosis. The problem was that very few physicians knew about the disease. Concentrations of cholesterol in blood plasma were not generally measured, and the patients usually have no symptoms before their first heart attack, which can often be fatal. Physician inexperience with familial hypercholesterolemia is one of the most important reasons that the cholesterol controversy could continue for so many years.

Autopsy

The autopsy has taught us more about atherosclerosis than any other method of science. Leonardo da Vinci used it surreptitiously, and it has been at the center of atherosclerosis research in the 20th century.[5] The International Atherosclerosis Project was the first of a series of large autopsy studies organised by researchers at Louisiana State University in New Orleans. From 1960 to 1964 they looked at more than 23,000 sets of aortas and coronary arteries from autopsied persons in 14 countries, and they found that about 60% of the inner surface of coronary arteries was, on average, affected by advanced atherosclerosis in patients who had had symptoms of coronary heart disease. In contrast, in persons of the same age who had died for other reasons including accidents, the extent of artery surface affected by advanced atherosclerosis was 3%–17% in those aged 35–44 increasing to 11%–38% in those aged 65–69 years of age The same study showed that coronary atherosclerosis was significantly related to concentrations of blood cholesterol and to the percentage of calories that the person had eaten as animal fat.

Since it was apparent that atherosclerosis was usually the result of a very long process, the investigators in New Orleans initiated a series of cooperative studies of atherosclerosis in young Americans. They were carried out throughout the last quarter of the 20th century in collaboration with many other research groups. The most recent of the studies is called Pathological Determinants of Atherosclerosis in Youth. Abbreviated PDAY, it comprises nearly 3,000 persons aged 15–34, who had died by accident, murder or suicide. They were autopsied in forensic laboratories, and the extent of atherosclerosis in their arteries, measured by standardized methods, was related to blood cholesterol, smoking, blood pressure, etc. when they were still alive. It turned out that the extent of atherosclerosis in the coronary arteries and the aorta depended on how cholesterol was distributed among the various lipoproteins of the blood of the dead person. There was more atherosclerosis if the dead person had had a lot of cholesterol in LDL or in the lipoproteins that are converted into LDL (very low density lipoproteins (VLDL)). There was less if a lot of the cholesterol had been in high density lipoproteins (HDL). Cholesterol in LDL is often termed the "bad" cholesterol and that in HDL the "good" cholesterol. The amount of atherosclerosis also depended on whether or not the person had been a smoker and whether or not he or she had had high blood pressure.

These and several other autopsy studies confirmed once again that high cholesterol, smoking, high blood pressure and other risk factors for adult coronary artery disease speed up the formation of atherosclerosis already present in teenagers and in young adults, 20–30 years before coronary artery disease becomes clinically manifest. The studies provided explanations for data published many years previously, in 1953. That was the year the Korean War ended. It had begun in 1950, and during those four years about 54,000 Americans died on the Korean peninsula. Autopsies performed by military pathologists showed that 77% of young Americans killed in action already had coronary atherosclerosis.[6] The data caused a lot of concern at the time, because they confirmed suspicions about the increasing extent of coronary artery disease in the United States. The pathologists did not know for sure why the American soldiers, whose average age was only 22 years, had so much atherosclerosis, but they thought that diet might be important because, although they did not record how many young Koreans they studied, they noted that atherosclerotic plaques were rare in Koreans. They were also aware that LDL is higher in patients with coronary artery disease than in normal subjects, and they were aware of the possible importance of inflammation. Yet more than 40 years were to pass before most physicians were willing to consider lowering cholesterol in their patients to avoid the disease.

Population Studies

The Framingham Study was begun in 1948 to study, and monitor, the development of coronary heart disease in a group of middle-aged Americans living in Framingham in the state of Massachusetts. The Framingham Study and several other American as well as European epidemiological studies demonstrated that the incidence of coronary heart disease within and between populations increased as a function of concentrations of blood cholesterol, level of blood pressure and frequency of smoking.

By 1994, English epidemiologists could publish a review of 10 large cohort studies.[7] The term denotes a kind of population study in which investigators divide people into two or more groups (cohorts) according to whether, for one reason or another, they have been exposed to some factor thought to cause or prevent disease The groups are then followed long enough to determine the frequency of whatever might be the outcome of interest. The 10 cohort studies had recruited a total of nearly $\frac{1}{2}$ million men who sustained more than 18,000 episodes of coronary heart disease during the periods in which they were enrolled in the studies. The review, addressed at the cholesterol issue, showed that a modest 10% lower level of blood cholesterol was associated with an incidence of coronary heart disease which was 54% lower at age 40, 39% lower at age 50, 27% lower at age 60, 20% lower at age 70, and 19% lower at age 80. So, at all ages, the lower the cholesterol, the lower the risk, but benefits were greatest in the relatively young.

This kind of evidence is very suggestive, but it is not conclusive, and we shall return to the difference between evidence from observational studies and evidence from clinical trials in the chapter on evidence-based medicine. For the time being, let us look briefly at the history of the clinical trials of dietary and pharmacological treatments that have been directed at the cholesterol issue. In the early history of the drug trials we will find one of the reasons for the delay in accepting the cholesterol hypothesis of atherosclerosis, and in the more recent history of the drug trials, we shall find the most important reason that physicians ultimately accepted the same hypothesis.

Clinical Trials

In clinical trials, investigators allocate patients at random to two or more different kinds of treatment, placebo or active drug, for example, or control diet and intervention diet. Clinical trials are therefore methodologically more powerful than non-randomized cohort studies, in which the groups (the cohorts) can differ from each in many respects other than the one of interest.

The history of dietary trials has entailed some confusion, and the trials have been the subject of several, quite skeptical reviews.[8,9] It is therefore appropriate to emphasize how difficult it is to do good trials of dietary intervention. Food is complex, and it is impossible to change one component of food without changing at least one other. For example, if some of the saturated fat is removed from food it must be replaced by something else, usually carbohydrates (starchy food) or unsaturated fats in oils. If that isn't done, there will be loss of body weight because there is less energy in the food that is eaten. In either case, it can be difficult to know which change in food patterns has caused the effect observed (or not observed) in the results of the trial.

It must also be appreciated that these trials had to be done over many years, and there was no way that the researchers could be certain that people, as opposed to laboratory animals, did in fact eat the experimental food or the traditional food as they were supposed to. There was huge variation. It therefore makes sense to interpret the results of dietary trials within the context of the many other things that we know about food and disease, from physiology and observational epidemiology, and that overall interpretation usually results in the well-known recommendations about how to eat to reduce the risk of heart disease.

The early diet studies were quite naturally done to test an idea based on the results of epidemiological studies such as the Seven Countries Study. These epidemiological studies had shown that people who ate a lot of saturated fat from animals were more likely to be afflicted by heart disease than people who ate food with less saturated fat. It was therefore disappointing that trials of diets with a lower content of saturated fat, with a few exceptions,[10,11] did not produce very convincing evidence of a reduction of the occurrence of coronary heart disease. Somewhat more encouraging results were obtained from some but not all of the trials of vegetable oil supplements. The most encouraging results have come from two fairly small trials conducted in patients who already had coronary artery disease. Death rates were lowered very effectively in both of them. In the first this was due to eating fish or taking fish oil capsules,[12] and in the second it was due to a Mediterranean kind of diet with less saturated fat and more fats from both vegetables and fish.[12,13]

Taken together, the dietary trials show that there is no single component of food that unequivocally causes or prevents coronary artery disease. Removing only saturated fat, for example, will not do the trick, and just eating antioxidants will not do the trick. The trials also did not satisfactorily resolve the cholesterol issue. In fact, in both of the two trials showing the greatest beneficial effect of diet on risk of death, there was no appreciable effect on the concentrations of blood cholesterol.[12,13] Ultimately, the cholesterol issue was resolved by the drug trials, but here again there was a major problem.

The early clinical trials of the pharmacological lowering of cholesterol, published between 1975 and 1994, showed little reduction in the rates of heart attacks (myocardial infarctions) during the first two years of cholesterol reduction, but from year 2 to year 5, the average reduction in risk was 22%, and at 5 years it was 25%.[7] That may not seem so impressive, but considering that much more than half a century usually elapses from the appearance of the first signs of atherosclerosis in coronary arteries until death occurs by coronary heart disease, it actually had happened quite quickly. It can be appreciated as happening even more quickly if one recalls the point made in the previous chapter: in patients suffering end-point events, the duration of exposure to treatment with either placebo or active treatment is only one half of the length of a clinical trial. Most of the cholesterol-lowering trials lasted about five years, and patients who died or had myocardial infarctions had therefore been exposed to placebo or active drug for an average of only about $2\frac{1}{2}$ years. All in all, there was remarkable consistency between the results of the observational studies and the early clinical trials of lowering cholesterol. So what was the problem in the early trials?

The main problem was clofibrate. That is the name of one of the first drugs that could lower cholesterol effectively. In 1965, Michael Oliver in Edinburgh launched a gigantic clinical trial of treatment with clofibrate to see whether it could prevent coronary heart disease. The trial was performed under the auspices of the World Health Organization, and it included 10,267 men who had slightly elevated levels of cholesterol in their blood. Some of them lived in Edinburgh, others in Budapest and Prague. Half of them took clofibrate, and half of them took placebo for 5.3 years. Clofibrate lowered cholesterol by about 20%, and when the trial ended, it turned out that clofibrate also had reduced the rates of myocardial infarction and death by coronary artery disease by 20%. The problem was that clofibrate had increased deaths that had nothing to do with coronary artery disease. There was even some increase in cancer deaths.

The discipline of conducting clinical trials was not as well evolved then as it is now, and problems of methodology might have caused a spurious result. In any case, the increase in deaths observed in the trial was never adequately explained. Yet the results, published in 1978, caused physicians for nearly twenty years to be very skeptical of attempts to lower blood cholesterol by either drugs or diets.[14] There was widespread perception among them that lowering cholesterol was inherently dangerous, and, had it not been for the results of another major trial, the case for the benefits or otherwise of lowering blood cholesterol might have been closed forever. That trial was the LRC-CPPT, short for the Lipid Research Clinics' Coronary Primary Prevention Trial of a drug called cholestyramine.[15,16]

I still prescribe cholestyramine for a few of my patients, but it is not an easy drug to use. It is a powder that the patient must stir into water or orange juice before drinking it. It doesn't taste very nice, and it can cause constipation. In other respects it is a good drug, and it was used in the LRC-CPPT, an American trial of almost 4,000 men followed for more than seven years. It showed that the drug, given to half of the men, reduced the risk of fatal and non-fatal heart attacks by about 20%. There was no increase in total mortality. Those results persuaded pharmaceutical companies in the United States to invest in new drugs, and researchers to commit themselves to new trials, ultimately providing the evidence that allayed the concerns raised by the results of the WHO/clofibrate trial.

The new evidence was angiographic, x-ray images of the coronary arteries, and it was clinical, counting heart attacks and deaths among the participants. In more than 20 trials, coronary arteriography was performed in about 6,000 patients before and after reduction of blood cholesterol by diet, drugs or surgery. Most of these studies were published between 1984 and 1995. With the exception of the smallest of these trials, they all demonstrated, by one kind of measurement or another, that lowering cholesterol could inhibit the further progression of atherosclerosis in the coronary arteries. In several cases, some of the atherosclerosis even became less marked. These beneficial effects were statistically significant, but the anatomical improvements were in all cases so small that one would not expect that they could be of any clinical importance at all. It was therefore remarkable that clinical disease such as myocardial infarction was substantially reduced in most of these trials. Nevertheless, it required large trials of different statin drugs, employing many thousands of patients, to establish to everyone's satisfaction that cholesterol-lowering treatment is an effective and safe way to reduce the occurrence of coronary artery disease. The results of these six trials were published between 1994 and 2002. Together, they included more than 50,000 patients. Three of them were performed in patients who already had clinical coronary artery disease,[17–19] and two trials were done in persons without clinical coronary heart disease but at high or low risk of getting the disease.[20,21] The sixth included patients in both categories.[22] All six trials demonstrated that the lowering of cholesterol reduced risk of myocardial infarction, and in four of them the reduction in death rates was also statistically significant.

On the level of pathology and biochemistry there are several explanations for all of these findings. The most straightforward of them is that lowering the amount of LDL in the blood reduces the amount of cholesterol that gets into the artery wall. This allows the processes of removing cholesterol from the artery wall to get a chance to gain the upper hand. Another is that reduction of concentrations of LDL in the blood also reduces the amount of chemically modified LDL that gets into the wall of the artery. The result is that the artery wall is less inflamed. It cools off, and the atherosclerotic plaques in the wall therefore become less prone to rupture and to cause clotting of the blood. Yet another explanation is that cholesterol-lowering treatment makes the thin endothelial lining of the artery healthier so that the artery becomes less likely to contract in spasm. These explanations and several others are all supported by experimental data, and to varying degrees they probably all have a role to play in reducing risk, not only of having a myocardial infarction, but also of having a stroke.

The angiographic studies and the large clinical trials of statin therapy finally convinced physicians to take cholesterol seriously, and by the turn of the century many of them were taking statins to reduce their own risk of coronary artery disease.

Why Did It Take So Long to Draw Logical Conclusions From the Scientific Evidence?

The cholesterol question was resolved by all of this research and clinched by the statin trials. The effort took at least a half century. Why did it take so long? The documentation for lowering blood pressure in order to lower the risk of stroke and heart disease was no better, and neither the documentation for treatment of diabetes nor the documentation supporting cessation of smoking came anywhere close to the kind of evidence reviewed above. Yet treatment of diabetic patients to lower levels of blood sugar has been virtually without controversy, and there has also been much less controversy about treating high blood pressure. The controversies have concerned smoking and cholesterol.

I believe that there are two main explanations for the delay in accepting the cholesterol lowering hypothesis. One is that lowering cholesterol came to be perceived as being inherently dangerous. The other is that the cholesterol issue had become inextricably confused with larger issues concerning nutrition. In both cases, important concepts had become confused with each other, and the result was collective conceptual diplopia. Let's look at each explanation in turn.

Benefits of Cholesterol Lowering Depend on How You Do It

The WHO/clofibrate trial had created a problem: although clofibrate reduced the occurrence of coronary artery disease, it also seemed to increase overall death rates. The operation was a success, but the patient died. That result could have been due to a methodological flaw in the design or execution of the trial, but the real question was whether lowering cholesterol is inherently dangerous or whether clofibrate posed a danger unrelated to its cholesterol-lowering action.

In 1999, Swiss and Canadian researchers published a systematic review of the risk and benefit of different ways of lowering cholesterol.[9] The review comprised 59 trials that had involved more than 85,000 patients in the 59 treatment groups, and almost 88,000 patients in the 59 control groups. The ways of lowering cholesterol included treatment with statins and fibrates, but also treatment with other drugs such as resins, nicotinic acid, and hormones, and it included dietary intervention and treatment with fish oils.

The analysis included 12 trials of fibrates including the WHO/clofibrate trial. When all of the fibrate trial results were pooled, there was neither an increase nor a decrease in either the rates of death by coronary artery disease, the rates of death from other causes, or the rates of all deaths. As a class of drugs, the fibrates therefore seemed to be neither particularly dangerous nor particularly beneficial. Since the Swiss/Canadian analysis was performed, two other large fibrate trials have been published, one with a very positive result[23] and one with yet another equivocal result.[24] The results of the WHO/clofibrate trial, which contributed importantly to a twenty-year delay in efforts to lower blood cholesterol therefore did not seem to typify the fibrate trials. At the same time, though, the rest of the fibrate trials were unable to dispel all concerns about the utility of this group of drugs. All the King's horses and all the King's men could not put Humpty together again.

In contrast, the Swiss/Canadian analysis showed that the statin group of drugs reduced rates of death by coronary artery disease and rates of all deaths, whereas the rates of death from other causes were unaffected. Fish oils also reduced rates of all deaths, but the result was less robust than that of the statins, perhaps because the fish oil trials did not include nearly as many patients.

When the Swiss and Canadian investigators looked at all 59 trials at once, the variability in results could be explained largely on the basis of differences in the magnitude of cholesterol reduction. In other words, the reason that the statins were so effective in reducing deaths and deaths by coronary disease is that they are the most potent cholesterol-lowering drugs currently available. We can therefore finally be confident that lowering cholesterol is worthwhile, but that the way you do it does make a difference.

Food and Cholesterol

The second explanation for the delay in drawing the logical conclusions from the evidence linking cholesterol to coronary artery disease is that nutrition became the point of departure for the scientific and public debates. In contrast, the points of departure for understanding the importance of high blood pressure and high blood sugar were physiology, biochemistry and clinical experience.

Early on, cholesterol became inextricably associated with food, in particular with the meat and milk of our large domesticated mammals. Had focus instead been on genetics, biochemistry and clinical experience, I believe there would have been less controversy. This could have been the case if the point of departure had been familial hypercholesterolemia, just as the point of departure for treatment of patients with diabetes was type I diabetes, and the point of departure for treatment of high blood pressure was the dramatic disease called malignant hypertension. Type I diabetes is due to destruction of the cells of the pancreas that produce insulin, a mechanism entirely explainable in medical terms. In contrast, type II diabetes is due to overeating. Had type II diabetes been the point of departure for treatment of diabetic patients, I suspect it would have unleashed the same controversies as did treatment of patients with high cholesterol.

Patients with familial hypercholesterolemia do not attract the attention of physicians as well as do patients with diabetes, and the degrees to which physicians have been concerned with these two diseases differ enormously. There are reasons for this difference. Although type I diabetes is twice as common as familial hyper-cholesterolemia, it is in the same ballpark of prevalence. Approximately one in every 250 persons has type I diabetes, whereas one in 500 persons has familial hypercholesterolemia. With the exception of the rare patients with the homozygous form of famital hypercholesterolemia, moreover, patients with familial hypercholesterolemia are usually not as young as type I diabetic patients when they fall ill. Furthermore, while sudden death is often the first manifestation of familial hypercholesterolemia, the first symptoms of type I diabetes almost always bring patients to a hospital ward. The ratio of hospital units for diabetes and familial hypercholesterolemia is therefore much higher than two to one. For these reasons, the diseases identified with glucose were incorporated firmly into orthodox medicine, whilst the diseases identified with cholesterol were subjected to the vicissitudes of debate, medical and public. Familial hypercholesterolemia remained an erudite medical topic, and "cholesterol" became shorthand for the complicated relationship of animal fats to coronary heart disease.

The different points of departure for concern with cholesterol, blood pressure and glucose differed along the scale of severity of each condition. In general, the higher the cholesterol, blood pressure or glucose, the higher the degree of risk, but the relationships are not linear, and, as cholesterol, blood pressure or glucose steadily increase, the risk of disease increases ever faster. Moreover, high levels of cholesterol, blood pressure or glucose, and very high levels of risk, apply to very few people in any population. Most people have either normal or only slightly increased levels of cholesterol, blood pressure or glucose, and they have only slightly increased levels of risk. Since there are so many of them, however, most heart attacks and strokes occur in people who have been at only slightly increased risk and who have had only slightly increased levels of cholesterol, blood pressure or glucose.

Since type I diabetes and severely high blood pressure were the points of departure for concern with glucose and blood pressure, not only was the rationale not questioned, it also did not concern a large part of the population. Only later did type II diabetes and the less severe forms of hypertension attract much attention. In contrast, from the beginning, the cholesterol issue concerned nutrition rather than familial hyper-cholesterolemia. The focus was therefore on the large section of the population for which the major determinants of slightly elevated blood cholesterol are nutritional.

Benefits of treatment are greatest in patients at highest risk. For example, greater benefit is derived from reducing cholesterol from 8 to 6 mmol/l than from 6 to 4 mmol/l. The same applies to reducing blood pressure and blood sugar. Whereas the first trials of lowering blood pressure were performed in people with very high blood pressure, the first trials of lowering cholesterol by either diet or drugs were done in people with fairly low cholesterol levels such as the men in the WHO/clofibrate trial. The early clinical trials therefore demonstrated benefit to patients from lowering blood pressure but not from lowering cholesterol. Treatment of patients with severe type I diabetes was never subjected to a placebo-controlled trial because all physicians know that withholding insulin from such patients can be rapidly fatal. As yet there is also very poor evidence of benefit from treating patients with type II diabetes with drugs to lower blood sugar, but the poverty of that evidence has never had much impact on medical practice.

All this illustrates that medical tradition sometimes pre-empts the position usually accorded science. To a certain extent that's okay. There are other ways of knowing clinically important relationships than by reading the results of randomised clincal trials. A physician who has treated a patient acutely ill with malignant hypertension or a patient acutely ill with diabetic ketoacidosis will have been impressed by how sick these patients are and by the importance of treatment to lower blood pressure or blood sugar. There is no comparable condition associated with high blood cholesterol.

Intertwined with food, the cholesterol issue came to share the same fate as the tobacco issue. Both are cultural and economic issues. Smoking tobacco and eating animals are ingrained in many cultures, associated as they are with pleasure and a sense of predictability and security. Of the two, eating animals and animal products is ingrained more deeply than smoking. As we shall see in chapter 5, one of the ways of exploiting animals for food is in fact so old that it has had time to change the human genome in a small but important manner. Both issues concern agricultural products, and promotion of efforts to reduce consumption of tobacco and animal products have encountered sustained and sometimes bitter opposition from tobacco industry and food industry.[25]

There is a notable difference between the tobacco and food issues, however. The relationship of food to disease including coronary heart disease is not as straightforward as that of tobacco. Tobacco can afford pleasure and relaxation, but it has almost no redeeming qualitites in terms of health. In contrast, virtually all animal products are good sources of calories and protein, and they cause atherosclerotic disease only when too much is eaten for too long.

Because of the relatively simple connection between smoking and disease, representatives of the public health sector have won a partial victory over the tobacco industry in the United States, and the industry has shifted the focus of its marketing efforts to the developing countries. In contrast, there have been no advances in limiting the production of animals and animal products for food,[25] and it was not the food issue that settled the cholesterol issue. It was settled because the great drug trials of the 1990s and 2002 buried the concern created by the WHO/clofibrate trial. The later trials, moreover, bypassed the cultural problems posed by changes in eating pattens, and the cholesterol question was moved back into the realm of medicine and pharmacology. Divorced from the contentious issue of food, reduction of blood cholesterol by drugs became at once much more acceptable, not only to physicians, but also to patients.

Researchers who had provided most of the documentation until the beginning of the 1990s could never have done it on their own. The resolution of the cholesterol controversy ultimately required the help and resources of the pharmaceutical industry. The question is, of course, whether control of the epidemic of coronary artery disease of necessity also must be pharmacolgical.

Chapter 5

Food and Coronary Artery Disease

The food we eat and the air we breathe can make us sick or keep us well, and even school children know that eating fats, getting fat and smoking cigarettes cause heart disease. Exactly how eating and smoking do so is incompletely understood, but attention to dietary fat and avoidance of obesity and tobacco are justifiably at the center of all efforts to promote health in populations. The questions to be addressed in this chapter do not challenge that policy, but they concern some of the reasons why it is apparently so difficult to implement. Given the choice, why do so many of us eat too much, especially too much saturated fat?

On one level, the problem is behavioral: we know how to behave, but we don't want to. That dilemma can be couched in more dignified terms, and a whole science of behavioral medicine and whole institutions of various kinds of health workers have arisen to tackle it. Why misbehaviour is so pleasant is beyond my own expertise, but eating fatty and sugary food must be a deep desire, because it has spawned so many witticisms. They are mostly about food and death:

- Eat barbecue today; there isn't any in Heaven.
- Most suicides are committed with knife and fork.
- I don't want to be in too good shape if I get a terminal illness.
- Lipid-lowering diets don't make you live longer. They only make life seem longer.

A prominent British cardiologist was particularly fond of the last witticism, and it became part of the lore of medicine in the United Kingdom for several generations of physicians. He was wrong about the first half of the quip, but the second half was correct. To most people, food that lowers cholesterol doesn't taste as good as food that raises cholesterol. Is that the simple answer to a question that only academics find complicated?

Simple yes, but adequate no. Not only does fatty food taste good; it has also increased our chances of survival during the thousands of years of the formation of our genome. There are therefore several levels on which to understand choice of food when choice of food is possible. Apart from psychological and behavioral explanations, there are historical and genetic explanations, and this chapter is a brief discussion of these determinants of individual food choice. In the following chapter on agriculture I shall attempt to discuss some of the societal determinants of food availability.

Food and Coronary Artery Disease

Survival once depended upon the ability not only to obtain food but also to choose safe food. Such knowledge is less necessary now, but interest in food seems undiminished. Any journalist worth his salt can write about food as well as sex, war and kittens, and how to prevent heart disease by choosing the right food is staple stuff in weekly magazines. Many people know more or less perfectly which foods promote heart disease and which do not. A brief description of current dietary recommendations and their scientific rationale is therefore like preaching to the choir, but it is integral to the logic of the core thesis of this book: that coronary artery disease is a function of what we choose to eat (and smoke) among the products that farmers provide for us.

The nutritional determinants of atherosclerotic diseases are the objects of basic molecular biology and cell studies and experimentation on animals, but ultimately it is the results of observational and interventional epidemiology in humans that clinch the arguments for or against recommendations about what to eat. Comparisons of the consumption of food and the occurrence of coronary artery disease in different countries have shown that death by coronary heart disease is more common in populations which consume large amounts of animal products than in those which consume more vegetable foods. The prototype of this kind of cross-cultural study is the Seven Countries Study. In a report from that study, investigators described the association between the intake of major food groups and rates of death by coronary artery disease over a 25 year period in the USA, Finland, Holland, Italy, former Yugoslavia, Greece and Japan.[1] In general terms, death rates were higher in populations which were consuming large amounts of food from land animals, and they were lower in populations consuming large amounts of vegetables as well as fish and alcohol. When each food group was analyzed at a time (univariate analysis), high rates of consumption of butter, meat, pastries and milk were all related to increased deaths by coronary artery disease. The reverse pertained to legumes, oils, and alcohol: they seemed to lower risk of disease.

The results of cross-cultural studies are consistent with those of observational studies of nutrition and coronary artery disease performed within populations, and they are consistent with the results of trials of dietary intervention. Trials performed in patients with coronary artery disease, in particular, have shown that these patients live longer when meat, eggs, cream, hardened fats, including butter, are completely or partially replaced by fruits, vegetables, root vegetables, legumes, bread, nuts, fish, and fish oil or canola oil.[2–4]

Although some controversies remain there is, therefore, broad agreement between various authorities about most of the components of a diet that can be expected to reduce the risk of atherosclerotic disease.

Current Dietary Recommendations

In terms of the food choices that individuals must make, the recommendations are fairly simple. These are to eat plenty of vegetables, fruits and nuts, to eat plenty of whole grain, breads, rice and pasta, to eat lean meats and fish, and to use oils from olives, rapeseed, soy, maize, and sunflower. On the negative side the recommendations are to eat and drink fewer dairy products, less fat from pigs, cows and sheep, less coconut oil and palm oil, and less sugar, salt and alcohol. The fat in dairy products and meats, as well as the fat in coconut oil and palm oil, raises the blood cholesterol. Salt increases the blood pressure. And fatty and sugary foods and drinks, as well as alcohol, easily increase body weight. Obesity must be avoided. The obese must eat less and exercise more, and, of course, those who are not yet obese must avoid eating too much and exercising too little.

In biochemical terms, the picture that has resulted from the last few decades of research is more complex, but it is important to understand for administrators and politicians making decisions that affect population health. Many components of food affect risk, which is determined by some sort of collective action between them all, and a good diet is likely to protect patients from the consequences of atherosclerosis by several different mechanisms. They could involve not only protection against the accumulation of cholesterol in the artery wall but also protection against inflammation of the artery, oxidation of components of blood and the artery, thrombosis and coagulation, malfunction of the endothelial lining of the artery wall and disturbances of heart rhythm.

Of the many components of food involved in atherosclerosis, fats remain the best studied, and ultimately they may also remain the most important. Appendix 2 contains brief definitions of some of the technical terms used to describe different fats.

Only a few years ago, the main concern was the total amount of fat in food. That is the reason, of course, that so many items in grocery stores are labelled "low-fat". It is now apparent, however, that it is the type of fat rather than the amount of fat that affects risk of disease.[5] Among the many different kinds of fat, the prime culprits are saturated fats and trans-fats. Saturated fats are found mainly in dairy products and in the fat of the large mammals like pigs, cows and sheep. Palm oil and especially coconut oil also contain large amounts of saturated fatty acids (about 50% and 90%, respectively), and they are the exceptions to the general rule that vegetable fats are not saturated. A typical recommendation is that less than 10% of food energy should be from saturated fats.[6,7]

Trans-fats are unsaturated fats, but they have been "*trans*formed" in a way that makes them behave like saturated fats, in food as well as after uptake into the blood from the intestine. Trans-unsaturated fats are produced in the stomach of ruminant animals like the cow, and they get into the cow's mammary glands in the udder. So even though some of the fats of cow's milk are unsaturated, they are not of the healthy kind. Trans-unsaturated fats are also produced industrially as a by-product of the hydrogenation of the vegetable oils from which to make margarines. For technical reasons, industry considered them desirable until research showed that they were associated to coronary artery disease. They have now been removed from high-quality margarines, but they are still present in many fast foods. They are, for example, produced in vegetable frying oils, especially when the oils are used repeatedly. The amount of energy derived from trans-fats should be less than 2%[7] or as low as possible.[8]

When the amount of saturated fat is reduced in food, carbohydrates or other fats must replace it if the energy content of food is not to be reduced as well. Many of the controversies over diet have concerned the choice of substitute for saturated fat. In official recommendations, the emphasis on complex carbohydrates as a replacement for saturated fat has declined a little, and the recommendations are now for complex carbohydrates to contribute 55–60% of energy. The alternatives are polyunsaturated or monounsaturated fat, and results of the last two decades of research indicate that emphasis should be shifted from polyunsaturated to monounsaturated fats as replacement fats.[8,9] Most recommendations now feature a modest amount of polyunsaturated fat, up to 10% of energy, and a somewhat greater percentage of energy from monounsaturated fat, up to 20%.

The recommendations concerning the composition of polyunsaturated fats have also changed. The view that all polyunsaturated fats are beneficial, which was held 20–30 years ago, has now been abandoned, because we now know that there are important nutritional differences between them. Polyunsaturated fats from oily fish and certain vegetable oils, especially rapeseed and soy, are of the so-called *n*-3 variety, rather than of the *n*-6 or *n*-9 variety (see Appendix 2 for explanations), and it turns out that they have a variety of specific health benefits including lower risk of coronary artery disease and lower risk of sudden death. One recommendation is that a small amount of these *n*-3 fats (2 grams of α-linolenic acid and 200 mg of very long-chain fatty acids) should be eaten every day.[7]

Some of these recommendations are given in the table.

Outside of the small world of official recommendations, an important development based on the "low-fat" message has taken place in the real world of the consumer. The "low-fat" message has been exploited and misused by certain industries to sell enormous amounts of soft drinks and candies, especially to children, teenagers and young adults.[9] These products are certainly "low-fat", but they are energy-dense, and they are quite effective in making people fat. In fact, they are an important reason for the obesity epidemic that is spreading among our young people all over the economically developed world.

Percentage Distribution of Energy Intake in Different Recommendations

	Europe[6]	Europe[7]	USA[8]	Asia[10]
total fat	< 30%	< 30%	25–35%	< 21%
saturated fat	< 10%	< 10%	< 7%	
trans fat		< 2%	low	
monounsaturated fat	> 10%		up to 20%	
polyunsaturated fat	< 10%	4–8%	up to 10%	
complex carbohydrate		> 55%	up to 60%	

Official documents concerning prevention of cardiovascular disease include many other recommendations. The latest European recommendations, for example, stipulate that average intake of fruits and vegetables should be at least 400 grams/day, and that intake of salt (sodium chloride) should not exceed 6 grams/day.[7] Other recommendations concern cholesterol, fibre, plant sterols, soy protein, folate and other vitamins, potassium, calcium, and alcohol[7,8] and the reader should consult these documents for a full discussion and listing.

Before we leave recommendations and proceed to a discussion of the larger context of food and disease, a word or two about interactions. Smoking tobacco and possessing genes conducive to coronary artery disease result in disease mainly in populations in which people consume large amounts of dairy products and the meat of the large mammals. With few exceptions, it is the combination of circumstances that causes disease, not any one of them on its own. If you have not chosen your parents wisely, be sure to eat wisely. And if you smoke, you lessen risk of coronary artery disease, but not lung disease, by eating wisely.

And another word or two about further research. There are many links in the chain of events that leads from cause to effect. Cholesterol is just one of the elements necessary for arteries to become diseased by atherosclerosis. Many other but as yet unidentified links are probably as necessary, and removal of any one of them might also be sufficient to interrupt the causal chain. The utility of more research is that it might identify links that could be even easier to break than the cholesterol link.

Nevertheless, we already know a lot about what we should and should not eat to remain healthy. We know that in biochemical terms, and we know it as we move along the aisles in the supermarket. Yet, we continue more or less to choose the wrong items to place in the shopping cart. Why?

Food Preferences

Rats, pigs and humans are omnivores. All three of us, so to speak, must be able to figure out how to find nutritious food and how to avoid poisonous food. We are not specialist species that eat only one kind of food, grasses or insects for example. Throughout life we are presented with countless choices of food, and what we choose to eat is determined by our genes, by our culture and by our experience. The relative importance of these three determinants of food choice depends on the level of analysis: species, populations or individuals.

Almost by definition, genes are the most important determinants of food choice on the level of species, humans versus other animals. It takes a long time to make a genome, much longer than the history of our species and our immediate ancestors. But consider nevertheless some biologically recent time spans. The hominids departed from the other primates at least 6 to7 million years ago.[11] Homo erectus appeared about 1.7 million years ago. Early homo sapiens appeared about $\frac{1}{2}$ million years ago, and the history of humans proper took off between 100,000 and 50,000 years ago with the appearance of modern man (Cro-Magnon), the only remaining hominid after the disappearance of the Neanderthals about 35,000 years ago.

Plants and animals were probably first domesticated in the Near East, about 8500 B.C. and 8000 B.C. respectively.[12] Modern man has therefore spent more than 40,000, perhaps as much as 90,000 years as a hunter-gatherer and at most 10,000 years as a farmer. To the extent that our genome has been influenced by these systems of food acquisition, the hunter-gatherer period must have had a much greater effect on genetic determinants of food preference than the agriculturalist period, and studies of modern hunter-gatherer societies suggest that meat might have provided 65%, and gathered foods 35%, of the energy in the food of Paleolithic man.[13] However, genes affecting food preference, and many of the other ways we think and behave, must go back even further in time, easily to the appearance of homo erectus, but probably much farther back than that. We are likely to share any such genes at least with the anthropoid primates (chimps, gorillas and orang-utans), whose food is mainly vegetarian.[14] Thus, we don't really know what our genome wants us to eat, but fruits, vegetables and a little meat is a good guess. It probably does not particularly want us to eat grains or to drink milk after the first years of life.

One reason for uncertainty about the genetics of food preference, is that there has not been a huge field of research, to say the least. Nevertheless, a small number of studies have been done, mostly in affluent, white, middle-class American and Western European populations.[15,16] Strictly speaking, the results are therefore not necessarily applicable to other populations. If the genetics of food preference are as old as argued in the preceding paragraph, however, it is difficult to imagine that most of them are not shared by all humans. It seems likely that they pertain to the species rather than to different populations of humans. Examples are genetically determined preferences for sweet rather than bitter, for the known rather than the unknown, and for salt and fat.

Very young children have a taste for sweet food like human milk. They reject things that taste sour and bitter. Sensitivity to bitterness seems to be a heritable trait, and avoiding bitter things probably had survival advantages once, because bitterness often predicts toxicity. Avoiding bitter foods is less advantageous now, because many valuable vegetables can be bitter (e.g. citrus fruits and cruciferae like broccoli, cabbages, etc.). In an age of ready access to non-poisonous foods, sensitivity to bitterness could even be a risk factor for diet-related chronic disease.

Neophobia is another heritable trait affecting food choice that emerges at about two years of age. It can be a frustrating experience when a young child stubbornly refuses to eat something he has not tried before but which you know is good for him. If you are the parent or grandparent, however, congratulate yourself on having transmitted to him, or her, a constellation of genes for neophobia that once were vital. In fact, without those genes, you might not be having that particular frustrating experience at all, because the chain of ancestors leading down to you would have been interrupted by a little death when your would-be ancestor left the hut to put something interesting into his mouth that he should have avoided. Neophobia served a protective function when our genes were laid down thousands of years ago: most plants and animals are not edible, and many are poisonous.[15] The ability to remember the consequences of eating certain foods is as essential as neophobia. Rats have that ability, and so do we, and it must also have been worked into our genome long ago.

A preference for salt emerges in humans approximately 4 months after birth, and later in childhood we begin to like fatty food. Sodium appetite and hunger are, like thirst, also very likely to be genetically determined. A preference for fatty food, which contains a lot of energy, would have been useful when food supplies were scarce. In environments of food plenty, however, fatty food tends to make people fat, but men and women seem to differ in what they like to eat along with fat. Fat women prefer fat and sugar, whereas fat men prefer fat, protein and salt.

On the level of populations and individuals, as opposed to the level of species, genetic variation is probably a minor determinant of food choice. We know this from twin studies showing that the food preferences of identical twins do not differ very much from the food preferences of fraternal twins.[17] Instead, on these levels of analysis, cultural forces emerge as perhaps the strongest determinants of food choice, but they are integrated with personal experience, and with any possible individual genetic variation, into complex behaviours and a complex psychology of food preferences. The power of cultural influence is apparent to anyone living in multicultural societies. Generations after immigration, families tend to practice the cuisine their forefathers brought with them to the new country.

Of greatest importance for the prevention of coronary artery disease is that food choice, as opposed to food preference, can be powerfully influenced by family and, especially, by social forces. One such force is the explicit teaching of what should be eaten. Eat this, eat that, don't eat this and that! In families, parents teach their children what foods to eat, and on the social level promoters of population health do the same. As heart foundations hope, and as the food industry knows, it sometimes does work. The other is a complex of indirect social forces. They include, as examples, policies affecting taxation, agriculture, and food distribution, and they can determine which foods and beverages become more or less easily available.[9,17] That theme is central to this book.

Food Sources: Animals and Plants

Patterns of food consumption in the affluent societies of Western Europe and North America differ substantially from those pertaining to the time when the human genome was formed. In evolutionary terms, the change accompanying replacement of hunter-gatherers by farmers is quite recent, and evolution has probably not had time to take any notice at all of the change resulting from the emergence of modern affluent societies. Nevertheless, the recent history of numerous human diseases is closely linked to those transitions in food patterns. Coronary artery disease is just one of them.

Farming and the domestication of animals did not occur at once, but, measured along the scale of genetic evolution, they happened quickly. About 10,000 years ago, almost everyone lived on wild food. Eight thousand years later, almost everyone lived on food produced by farmers.[18] Most of us have probably been taught that the introduction of agriculture was an achievement of human cleverness, and in a sense it was, but historians now believe that it was driven by overpopulation. Hunting and gathering required a lot of space per human, and once human populations reached critical levels, which varied according to climate, vegetation, and fauna density, they were forced to adopt farming. In words not my own,[18] man had the choice of becoming celibate or clever, and, no surprise, he chose the latter.

During those 8,000 years of transition to farming, the story of this fundamental change of life must have been told and retold in countless versions. It seems to me that one of them might even have survived into our own religious literature as the story of the banishment of Adam and Eve. Adam had to eat the thorns and thistles and herbs of the field. *"In the sweat of thy face shalt thou eat bread"*, and Eve could no longer gather up fruits from the ground. Not to speak of plucking them from trees, of course. Good friends in theology say that I'm wrong about this, and that there is no evidence that Eden represents our past as hunters and gatherers. Still, the idea hasn't been proven to be wrong.

What seems certain is that farming also caused disease, and the average state of health seems to have deteriorated. The skeletons of neolithic farmers are typically some inches shorter than the skeletons of their ancestors, the paleolithic hunter-gatherers.[19] The causes of the poorer health of farmers were nutritional and infectious diseases. The food of hunter-gatherers was (and is) extremely varied, consisting mainly of fruits, vegetables and meat. In contrast, farming communities quickly became dependent on one or a few staple crops. The result could be frequent deficiencies of vitamins or protein.

Pellagra, due to lack of the vitamin niacin, is a good example. It causes diarrhoea, dementia and death, and it is due to dependency on maize as a staple crop. Similarly, beri-beri, a disease of the nervous system and the heart, is due to lack of vitamin B1 (thiamine). It occurs in populations dependent on rice, when the rice is stripped of the husk that contains vitamins including thiamine. We succumb to scurvy, as yet another example, if we do not get vitamin C, and our inability to synthesize that simple molecule is one more piece of testimony to a past as hunters and gatherers when we ate so many fruits and vegetables that we didn't need to make the vitamin ourselves.

Deficiency of protein was a disease of early farmers, and kwashiorkor continues to be a serious problem in the developing world. Children become stunted when when they are weaned from breast milk to a cereal pap containing inadequate protein. *Kwashiorkor* is an African word meaning the *"sickness of the deprived child"*.[18] The great infectious diseases of man have also been thought to be the result of agriculture and the domestication of animals. Historians estimate that humans share about 65 diseases with dogs, 50 with cattle, 46 with sheep and goats, 42 with pigs, 35 with horses, and 26 with poultry. For example, smallpox is probably the result of a long process of adaptation of cowpox to humans, and the various forms of influenza come from pigs, birds and horses. Measles may be the result of rinderpest in cattle and canine distemper in dogs. Humankind has now lived with these viral diseases for so long that large parts of the human genome are viral in origin. Viruses, bouncing back and forth between us and the animals sharing our houses and farms, have indelibly marked our genome.

Other infectious diseases due to agriculture are not viral. Irrigation farming allowed, for example, the emergence of schistosomiasis, a debilitating and sometimes deadly disease due to a parasitic worm that, in certain stages of its life cycle, requires a snail living in paddies and irrigation canals as a host. It is common now in developing countries, and it has been found in the kidneys of 3,000 year old Egyptian mummies. The parasite that causes malaria, which is believed to have originated among African primates, also needs an intermediate host, the Anopheles mosquito. The mosquito breeds extensively in cultivated lands with ponds and paddies.

The origins of human infectious diseases are not only agricultural, of course, and the agricultural explanation, as popularised by Jared Diamond,[12] is a simplification.

Molecular studies of the phylogeny of micro-organisms have become possible during the last decade of the 20th century. They have shown, for example, that dysentery and tapeworm diseases, once thought to have been acquired during the domestication of animals, must have been with us for much longer.[20] Nevertheless, the forced abandonment of life as hunters and gatherers for a life as farmers was probably the single most important determinant of the history of human diseases, and it had implications beyond human health.

Kenneth F. Kiple writes that "it was from this crucible of the agricultural revolution that people began learning to manipulate the planet — to rearrange its ecological systems, not to mention the genes of the plants and animals within those systems. They began the enterprise of undoing a self-regenerating nature without knowing what they were doing, an unthinking process that has continued to the present".[18]

The changes in patterns of food consumption caused by the recent transition from traditional farming societies to present-day affluent societies are of a different kind, but they have been almost as great as those resulting from the transition from hunter-gathering to agriculture. Labarthe argues that the more recent changes have, in fact, been even greater, at least in terms of the major nutrients of food.[21] Intake of protein declined a little from 15%–20% of energy to 10%–15% when peasant agriculturalists replaced the hunter-gatherers. Sugar had previously not been a part of human diet, but it came to provide about 5% of energy. In modern affluent societies, protein intake has declined further to 12% of intake, whereas sugar has increased further to 20%. As strikingly, intake of fat has increased from 15%–20% in hunter-gatherer societies and 10%–15% in peasant agricultural societies to 40% or more in modern affluent societies. These increases have been at the expense of starch. In compositional terms, fat intake has doubled, salt has increased by a factor of 10, and intake of sugar has increased from 0% to 20%. To compensate, intake of energy as starch and fiber has been halved.

For most populations, or for the major proportion of any one population, the change from the food of a peasant agriculturalist to a modern affluent society has occurred within the last 150 years. The changes in the food of the Englishman, discussed in Chapter 2, are well documented examples. It should be emphasized, however, that even the English data are averages, and certainly the overall data do no justice to the cultural, temporal and geographical diversity of the history of what we eat. This is particularly important in the long term, because long term differences between populations in availability of different foods can have produced genetic differences.

The Relationship of Genes to Environment

Charles Darwin provided us with the first consistent view of how plants and animals have evolved. As mutations occur at a fairly constant rate throughout the genomes of plants and animals, successive generations of any given variety or species of plants and animals gradually change. Sometimes these genetic changes make the plants or animals better or worse suited to survive in their environment. Those better adapted to the environment tend to survive and to pass their modified genes on to later generations. Darwin did not know about genes, and he did not write about mutations. Instead, he wrote about the innumerable slight variations and modifications in all varieties of plants and animals that over time gradually accumulate to differentiate progeny from progenitors, but most of his thinking was perfectly consistent with modern biology.[22]

Our own genome has evolved down along the chain of life from ancestor species not resembling us very much at all. A community of primitive cells, if not a single kind of bacterium, is believed to be the ancestor of all living things.[23] Now finally human, our genome has been sculpted by the interaction between us, or our animal predecessors, and our ever changing environments through several billion years. In thinking about environments, emphasis has shifted from the concept of adaptation of living organisms to environments to the concept of interaction between organisms and environment.

In traditional Darwinian thinking, environment is independent of the living organisms within it, and organisms must perish or find a way to adapt to it. That particular Darwinian concept is clearly wrong, however. Richard Lewontin of the Museum of Comparative Zoology at Harvard University argues that all organisms actively construct, in the literal sense of the word, a world around themselves, and they are in a constant process of constructing and altering their environment.[24] Nests are part of the environment that birds build for their chicks, and urban humans live in environments largely constructed by themselves. In this there is nothing new, says Lewontin. Even the composition of the air in which we live is a consequence of ancient biological processes. The pre-biotic atmosphere contained very little free oxygen; most of the oxygen was in carbon dioxide. The oxygen of our present atmosphere was made by photosynthesis in ancient plants, which also trapped the carbon dioxide. In other words, our life depends on an atmosphere that could not have come into existence except as a product of the organisms that were our very distant ancestors. The dualism of genes and the environment is therefore misleading. Evolution of new life forms has taken place in a constant interaction between genes, organisms and the environment.

Man has fashioned his environment as much as any animal. He has even created environments to which he later has become genetically better adapted. The classic example is the protection against malaria enjoyed by bearers of a mutation in the gene for the globin part of haemoglobin in the red cells of blood. The mutation causes sickle cell anaemia, but you have to have the mutation in both of your two versions (alleles) of the gene (one from each parent) to get the anaemia. If you have the mutation in only one of your two versions of the gene, a much more common condition, you don't get anaemia, and you also happen to be protected against malaria. About 80 million people are protected in this way. They are inhabitants or descended from inhabitants of warm or temperate regions of the world where the conversion of forests to farmland had created drainage and irrigation ditches, water holes and puddles. Here the Anopheles mosquito could thrive. Sometimes the mosquito is infected with the protozoan parasite that causes malaria when the mosquito injects it into humans by biting them. By selection, some people thus acquired a genetic variation that protected them from the consequences of the mosquito bite, itself a consequence of man's adoption of life as an agriculturalist.

Lactase Persistence and Thrifty Genes

Another example of genetic adaptation in humans to an environment created by humans is more pertinent to this book, because it is conducive to coronary artery disease. It is lactase persistence, perhaps the most important single genetic determinant of risk of coronary artery disease. It also has to do with farming, survival and, perhaps, conquest.

Man first domesticated animals in the Fertile Crescent of the Middle East about 10,000 years ago, slightly later perhaps in China, and probably much later in Africa, New Guinea and the Americas. Jared Diamond has popularised the argument that farming and the domestication of large animals enabled the Eurasians in particular to build complex states capable of subjugating their neighbours.[12] Complex states could arise only when many people could be liberated from the work of producing food so that they could become craftsmen, bureaucrats and soldiers instead. Large domesticated animals could pull plows, and some of them could pull chariots or carry warriors on their backs.

As we noted a little earlier in this chapter, animals provided agriculturalists, Eurasians especially, with other assets as well. Smallpox, chickenpox, mumps, measles, influenza, tuberculosis, cholera, malaria, plague, and yellow fever are thought to have evolved from diseases of animals. When we live close to animals, we must share viruses, bacteria and other micro-organisms with them, and parasites find a way to force themselves, as unwelcome guests, upon both animals and humans hosts at some time in their own life cycle. We get the bugs of animals, and they get ours. Although infectious diseases made dreadful inroads into urban populations, frequent exposure ensured varying degrees of immunity and sometimes genetic adaptation. Europeans, especially, could travel to other regions of the world as carriers of germs that were lethal mainly to other peoples. The Spanish conquistadores were *"immunological supermen"*, because the Atlantic and Mediterranean seaports of the Iberian peninsula had *"served as clearing-houses for swarms of diseases converging from Africa, Asia and the Americas"*.[19] Infectious diseases were the biggest killers of American Indians in the 16th and 17th centuries and of Native Australians in the 19th century.

The Europeans also brought with them the ability to tolerate the milk of domesticated mammals. That ability is lost by most other humans in early childhood, and by all other land mammals at the time of weaning. At that time in life, activity of lactase, an enzyme in the cells lining the small intestine, drops to 10% or less. Lactase is necessary to break down lactose, or milk sugar, so that its component parts can be absorbed into the blood stream. Drinking milk after the normal involution of intestinal lactase can elicit vomiting and diarrhoea as well as abdominal pain and distension, because lactose reaches the large intestine (the colon), where it is fermented by bacteria. Production of carbon dioxide and short chain organic acids by fermentation causes abdominal discomfort. The involution of intestinal lactase function serves a clear purpose in the life of animals and the survival of species, since it helps to ensure that weaning takes place. Animals unable to wean their young would not survive very long in the wild.

Europeans as well as several peoples in Africa, the Near East and India are able to tolerate milk after childhood because the lactase in their intestine remains active.

Persistence of enzymatic activity is probably due to a mutation in a gene normally responsible for turning off lactase. It is easy to understand how that mutation could have conferred advantages in the special setting of agricultural and nomadic societies. Frederick J. Simoons of the University of California-Davis, proposed that in times of food scarcity, persons with lactase could drink milk, or they could drink more milk than others. That enabled them to exploit not only milk sugar but also milk fat and milk protein.[25] In countries far to the north, the calcium derived from milk might also have offset a tendency to rickets and osteomalacia due to deficiency of vitamin D, which is produced in the skin when it is exposed to sunlight. K. David Patterson believed that the mutation causing lactase persistence probably occurred independently in northern Europe and in the nomad populations of Arabia, Sahara and eastern Sudan, where lactase persistence increased human ability to exploit camels and cattle in a harsh and arid environment.[26] And, of course, since the milk everywhere was from animals, not women, lactase persistence did not interfere with weaning.

The cover illustration for this book is a photograph of the Ymer Well by the Danish sculptor, Kai Nielsen. He unveiled the sculpture in 1913, and it shows Ymer suckling at the udder of the cow, Audhumbla. According to Nordic mythology, Ymer was one of the ancient giants who were vanquished by the Nordic gods. The gods then created the cosmos from Ymer's body. His cranium became the firmament, his blood became the rivers and the oceans, and so on and so forth. The reader will appreciate that the Scandinavians of about a thousand years ago considered Ymer very ancient indeed, and the Ymer Well illustrates, in stone no less, our belief in the antiquity of our connection to domesticated animals and their milk. In Denmark, yoghurt is called "*ymer*". The sculpture is very well done, but in 1913 it caused a scandal, in part because of Ymer's large genitals. Kai Nielsen probably did not equate them with genetics, but the magnificent size of Ymer's genitals certainly made it clear that he had matured past the age of normal weaning. Robustness, if anything, characterized Nordic mythology.

The ability to tolerate lactose can be measured by a biochemical test (breath test). The proportion of a population that tolerates lactose runs the gamut from almost 100% in northern Europe to nearly zero in Thailand. Populations with high proportions (61%–99%) are mainly northern Europeans and Americans of European ancestry. Populations with intermediate proportions are mainly southern Europeans, Hispanics and Black Americans, Turks, southern Indians, and Greenland eskimos (19%–66%), and populations with low frequencies (0% to 17%) are Asians including Chinese and Japanese, native Australians, natives of Papua New Guinea, Amerindians, African Blacks and Melanesians.[27] This distribution of the gene for lactase persistence makes sense if the mutation began to confer selective advantage about 400 generations ago (10,000 years), and parents with high lactase activity produced 1%–3% more children each generation than lactase-deficient parents.[28]

One or more mutations could cause lactase persistence, and they could have occurred more than once in human history. Lactase persistence in populations such as the Inuit (Eskimos) and the American Indians is, however, almost certainly due to interbreeding with Europeans.[29] At one point it was thought that lactase activity could adapt itself to large amounts of milk, but this so-called induction hypothesis is not compatible with most data, and researchers seem to agree that genes determine whether lactase stops functioning or not.

Consumption of milk products varies enormously across the planet, broadly conforming to the distribution of lactase persistence. In the developed countries of Europe and North America, for example, the average person consumed almost 200 kg of milk per year in 1990, whereas in China and Japan it was less than 7 kg.[30] The correspondence between lactase persistence and milk consumption is less than perfect for several reasons, however. First, the lactose content of milk can be reduced by fermentation or by the removal of the water phase as in the making of cheese, so that many people without lactase in adult life nevertheless can consume such modified dairy products. Secondly, people of European heritage are convinced of the benefits of milk, and they strongly urge people without lactase to drink it. For example, American Indian school children drank substantial amounts of milk in spite of symptoms of lactose intolerance.[29]

A third reason is connected to medicine. There is now greater recognition of the symptoms of lactose intolerance, and, as could be anticipated, the problem has been turned upside down. Lactase persistence is defined as the normal state, and the usual condition of most non-Europeans and all other land mammals is defined as a disease state. The "disease" is called lactose intolerance and even lactase deficiency. Although the inability to tolerate milk is of greater concern to the dairy industry than it is to physicians, tablets containing lactase are available as over-the-counter drugs. It is also possible to eat bacteria that can make lactase. The bacteria are introduced into the intestine by adding them to food as a dietary supplement (probiotic). In the intestine, the bacterial lactase breaks down lactose, and a person whose own lactase has been turned off can once again drink the milk of cows or other mammals.

Researchers have even developed animal models in which to study gene therapy for lactose intolerance. Let us look at these gene therapy experiments a little more closely. Like all other mammals, rats have little or no lactase function after weaning. The researchers inserted the lactase gene into a virus, and by feeding the virus to rats, they were able to get the gene into some of the cells of the intestine. That enabled these adult rats to regain the ability to break down lactose in the gut.[31] The researchers wrote that their data indicate that a "gene in a tablet" or a "genetic pill" might be useful for a broad range of conditions including lactase deficiency, *the world's most common genetic disorder, afflicting more than 50% of the world's population*.

The concept of gene therapy for more than half of mankind is breathtaking indeed. The article was published in a prestigious scientific journal, and there is no reason to think that it was not meant seriously. The research described could be viewed as an example of the perversion of science, but it is probably more fair to say that in science as well as in other human activities, the right hand doesn't necessarily know what the left hand is doing. The authors emphasized that the condition they sought to correct afflicted all mammals with the exception of about half of all humans, but there was no indication in the article that the authors had considered the possibility that lactase persistence could be seen as an abnormal state.

Nor did the authors mention coronary artery disease. Given the association of coronary heart disease with use of dairy products, however, it is no surprise that lactase persistence is roughly correlated with a high frequency of coronary heart disease. Annual age-standardised rates of death by coronary heart disease are about 300 per 100,000 in Europe and the USA, where approximately 80% of the population have persistent lactase function. In contrast, rates are about 175 per 100,000 in Japan and China, where about 10% of the population have persistent lactase function. Strictly speaking, these data prove nothing, but they are consistent with the idea that lactase persistence is part of the complex of conditions that promote coronary heart disease.

The persistence of lactase function is probably a genetic adaptation to easy access to milk of domesticated animals, conferring survival advantages in harsh environments. In more benign environments, lactase persistence could be a genetic determinant of the acceptability of one major source of animal fat and protein that promotes coronary heart disease. Since it is so common in many populations, it may be one of the most important genetic determinants of coronary artery disease.[32]

Lactase persistence is not the only example of a genetic variation that could be advantageous when food is scarce but disadvantageous when food is plentiful. A more celebrated example is the "thrifty gene". It is a concept rather than a gene, however. No single gene has as yet been unambiguously identified as being particularly thrifty. The concept, as first suggested by James V. Neel in 1962, was that insulin in people with thrifty genes worked very rapidly to prevent loss of sugar into the urine. Sugar, or glucose, contains energy, and in situations of frequent food shortage it was probably important to conserve as much energy as possible. Neel wrote that thrift in the use of energy would have been "*an asset to our tribal, hunter-gatherer ancestors with their intermittent, sometimes feast-or-famine alimentation*".

The original concept of the thrifty gene proved untenable as more became known about the physiology of insulin, but it survived in a more general form. It has, for example, been thought to apply to the Pima Indians of New Mexico. They were recently a neolithic people, but north of the Mexican-American border they now lead a life similar to that of other Americans. It is sedentary, and there is more than adequate food. The result is that many Pima Indians are very obese, and they are therefore also commonly afflicted by type II diabetes. The idea is that the obesity and type II diabetes of the Pima Indians both result from an exceptional, genetically determined ability to conserve energy in the form of fat. Obesity and type II diabetes are both associated with the early onset of coronary heart disease, and both conditions are also prevalent in Saudi Arabia, where natives were desert nomads just one or two generations ago.

Pima Indians and Arabians could both have genetic variations that permit them to conserve energy efficiently. They are not necessarily the same ones, however. A year before he died, James V. Neel published a revised version of his thrifty genotype hypothesis.[33] He wrote that there could be many different patterns of variation in several or many different genes, and each pattern (genotype) could enable the person to conserve energy efficiently. It is wrong to consider such genetic variations abnormal, however. Instead, "*. . . the genes involved are very predominantly fine old genes . . . honed by millennia of selection for harmonious interactions, . . . the proper functioning of which is overwhelmed*" by a new environment of food plenty and physical inactivity. Those genetic variations are abnormal only in the setting of food patterns that are very unusual in human history, and those patterns of eating exceed what our ancient genome can cope with.

We can always use more knowledge about food, and more research is certainly welcome, but existing knowledge is adequate for the prevention of coronary artery disease. If you were a visitor from another planet, however, you could not know that from watching us ordering food in cafeterias and restaurants or buying it in supermarkets. If we are affluent enough, we eat foods of a kind and quantity that will expand and maintain the disease in epidemic proportions. Some of the reasons for doing that are rooted in our own experience, in our culture, and in our genes.

In the next chapter we shall look more closely at the consequences of the structure of agriculture, and of agricultural policy, for food choice. Experience and culture are not easily amenable to policy decisions, and most of our genes are fine as they are. But the availability of different foods can be changed by agricultural and nutritional policy, and such change could assist us as individuals in making intelligent food choices. If that is not done, intelligence is up against an impressive array of forces unfavorable to habits of eating that promote human health.

Chapter 6

The Agricultural Connection

A sense of the history and structure of farming is helpful in understanding the relationships between human disease and agriculture that I attempted to discuss briefly in the previous chapter. This chapter will therefore take us further into subject areas that many nurses, physicians and managers and ministers of health care probably would not consider matters of medical concern, but I hope to show that consideration to be wrong.

I shall attempt to argue that some of the most widely held tenets of agronomical and medical biotechnology are less likely to help us to develop effective, sustainable and ecologically sound methods of feeding the world and preventing disease than less fancy solutions based on a more sophisticated understanding of the biology of farming and medicine. On the political level, I want to argue that we are not being serious about health care policy if we do not seek to understand what our neighbors in the schools of agronomy and in the ministries and departments of agriculture are thinking and planning. As a corollary, I argue that the effects of farming, not only on the environment, but also on human health, must be more explicitly entered into the formulation of agricultural policy. Others have advanced this argument more completely and more elegantly than I, but that emerging literature is virtually unknown to those of us who work in medicine.[1,2]

A Bit of History

As discussed in the previous chapter, meat was an important part of the food of hunters and gatherers, but animals were first domesticated only about 10,000 years ago, and the mass production of animals and animal products for consumption by whole populations of humans has happened only during the past 150 years. That development has been necessary for the epidemic of atherosclerotic disease to occur, and some of the major barriers to prevention of atherosclerotic diseases are encased in that history. It is beyond the scope of this book, and certainly beyond my abilities, to write the history of agriculture, but, drawing primarily on an analysis by the Danish historian, Thorkild Kjærgaard,[3] I shall try to suggest outlines of that history in a way to indicate why coronary heart disease has been and continues to be so difficult to eradicate. The sketch concerns the history of European agriculture since the 14th century, because that history indicates the trajectory along which North American agriculture and later the agriculture of the developing world, for better and worse, now are supposed to be progressing.

By the early 14th century, populations in Europe had grown to the point where much forest had been felled so that the land could instead be used for pasture and crops. The continent was beginning to suffer from the effects of overpopulation. That problem disappeared quite suddenly in 1347–1351, when the Black Death killed about 25 million people, or about a third of the population of western Europe. This demographic regression gave the forests of Europe a long respite from the axe and saw, but in the beginning of the 17th century the population of Europe was again increasing, and deforestation was resumed to clear land and to use wood for fuel, manufacture and building, not least for military purposes. The wars of the 16th and 17th centuries, especially the Thirty Years War of 1618–1648 in central Europe, required huge amounts of timber for land armies and for fleets of war ships. As an example, the area of Denmark covered by forest fell from the 20%–25% in 1600 to only 8%–10% in 1750.

By the middle of the 18th century, it was apparent that Europe was entering a new period of ecological crisis. Deforestation caused erosion of soil and flooding of land by a variety of mechanisms including the clogging up of rivers by silt and sand and reduced evaporation of water from trees. The result was increasing areas of desert, moorlands and swamps, that were no longer able to sustain agriculture. It was the Age of the Enlightenment, however, and enlightened use of technology saved Europe from ecological catastrophe, which would otherwise have occurred probably no later than 1830.

In many parts of eighteenth century Europe, farming was done on the great estates of the aristocracy. Later vilified by the victors of the 19th century political upheavals, most aristocrats had two attributes unrelated to whether they were scoundrels or not. They were educated, first of all. Aristocratic sons were schooled in a variety of disciplines including agronomy, which was well represented in the libraries of typical estates. Secondly, aristocrats had evident self-interest in the long term care of the lands that they were to pass on to their children and grandchildren. Ability and self-interest ensured good husbandry. In his history of Europe,[4] Norman Davis writes:

> Gentlemen were absorbed by the rising science of estate management, convinced that their properties could not simply be put in order but could be transformed into thriving businesses. Land reclamation by the Dutch or on the Dutch model changed the face of several low-lying regions, from the fenlands of East Anglia to the delta of the Vistula.

These landlords and the monarchs, some of whom were invested with "absolute power", agreed on a series of measures to avert ecological disaster. Where necessary, soil erosion was checked by extensive building of windbreaks and planting of forests, and flooding was controlled by dams and drainage. Soils could be improved on an empirical basis. Acidic, lime-deficient soils were improved by marling, and nitrogen was added by the sowing of plants of the pea family. Alfalfa was used mainly in southern Europe, whereas clover, probably introduced into Spain in the 13th century, had spread gradually into northern Europe by the early 18th century. In coastal areas, sea weed was another source of nitrogen.

Coal and iron could now be mined and exploited directly and indirectly as effective substitutes for wood. Coal provided fuel for the heating of houses, the burning of bricks, and the forging of iron, e.g. for shoeing horses and making stronger plows. The appearance of coal and iron in 18th century European agriculture signified industrialization, and it foreshadowed one of the most important characteristics and problems of agriculture at the opening of the 21st century: the dependency on fossil fuels.

In 1800, however, fossil fuel had contributed to the recovery of European agriculture, forests and biodiversity. From the middle of the 18th century, the number of species of plants and animals increased and peaked in 1820–1850. This recovery can be attributed to the huge undertaking organized not least by the aristocracy, which was repaid for its trouble by displacement from power, swiftly by the populace in France and later in Italy, or more slowly by the monarch and his public servants, as in the German states, Great Britain and Scandinavia. Considered within this perspective, the industrialization of agriculture, a prerequisite for the later epidemic of coronary artery disease, began about 50 years before the advent of the steam engine and 150 years before the advent of the internal combustion engine. In 1776 it was on Thomas Jefferson's farm in Virginia when he wrote the *Declaration of American Independence* (from Great Britain), and also when Edward Jenner made the connection between atherosclerosis of the coronary arteries, on the one hand, and angina pectoris and sudden death, on the other.

Despite differences, European and North American agriculture in the 19th century shared two advantages. First, the land was fertile, in Europe because of the developments just depicted, in North America because of the same developments in the early colonies. In the rest of the North American continent the land had, with rare exceptions, not been used for farming by the Indian population of mainly hunters and gatherers. The top soil was still there; farmers had not yet depleted it of nutrients and minerals.

Secondly, the same technology gradually became available to farmers in both Europe and North America. Increasingly effective farming machinery, powered by animals and later by fossil fuels, was introduced during the 19th and 20th centuries; artificial fertilizers became common from the middle of the 19th century; and throughout the period, systems for the transport and distribution of materials for farmers and produce from farms by railroads and trucking became more efficient and complex.

Rates of industrialization, not only of agriculture, differed substantially country by country. In 1750, the per capita levels of industrialization were approximately the same in Europe and in the American colonies as they were in Russia, China and India. By 1830, however, the British were for many reasons far ahead of all other countries, including those of continental Europe, and they maintained their lead into the 20th century. By 1913, however, just before the First World War, the United States had overtaken them. Great Britain was trailed by Belgium, Germany and France. Slower to industrialize were Austria-Hungary, Italy and Russia. Outside western Europe and North America, countries even de-industrialized. In 1913, China and India were behind their own 1750 levels,[5] and the Bolshevik Revolution in 1917 also reversed Russian industrialization.

The countries of Europe therefore necessarily exploited the potentials of industrialized grain production at different rates and in different ways. Whereas England and France elected to increase production of grains, especially wheat, Germany, Holland and Denmark elected to import grains from the Ukraine and the Americas for animal feed. Railroads and large ships made that transport feasible, and raising animals was more remunerative for farmers than raising grain. Mass transportation of fertilizers, grains, livestock and foods by water, rail and roads has since then become a hallmark of modern agriculture.

Modern Agriculture

The amount of manure obtained from animals limited the amount of crops that could be raised in traditional agriculture. With artificial fertilizers, much higher yields became possible, and artificial fertilizers enabled farmers to separate the raising of crops from the raising of livestock. Artificial fertilizers could theoretically have made it possible to create a vegetarian society without coronary heart disease, but that was not an objective of agricultural policy. Quite the contrary. Twentieth century agricultural policies as well as market forces have artificially linked the production of grains closely to the raising of livestock.

In the United States after World War II, farmers could raise more grain than was needed. Accordingly, taxation was used to increase the market for grains by encouraging farmers to raise livestock in feed lots rather than on pasture. Feed lots are enclosed plots of land without a blade of grass in which cattle might spend most of their lives, moving slowly about in their own manure. The feed is grain, and the result is a substantial increase in the production of meat, which gets fatty and, as we are taught, attractively marbled. It doesn't very much resemble the meat eaten by hunters and gatherers. American policies also affected agriculture in other countries, because the establishment of feed lots was tied to foreign assistance programs with the purpose of increasing the market for surplus American grain.[6]

Considerations of another kind entered into the formulation of European agricultural policy. Famine was part of a common European memory. The great famine of 1921–1922 in Russia, a consequence of the Bolshevik policies of requisitioning agricultural produce from peasants, resulted in about 5 million deaths.[7] Famines also occurred in many European countries during and after World War II. The main purposes of the Common Agricultural Policy, as stipulated in article 39 of the Treaty of Rome of 1957, were accordingly to increase agricultural productivity, to stabilize markets and to assure farmers of a reasonable standard of living and consumers of adequate food at reasonable prices.[8] Mechanisms initially employed to achieve these objectives were taxation of agricultural products imported into the European Union, subsidization of exports from the EU, and guaranteed minimum prices for agricultural produce within the EU. If European prices dropped below the guaranteed minimum price, farmers could sell their produce to the EU, which then would try to export it or dispose of it through free food schemes. The policy nevertheless resulted in huge surpluses of grains, meat and dairy products, which were later reduced as a result of reforms enacted in 1992, shifting the emphasis from price support to production control and direct payments to farmers (MacSharry Reform).

By these different mechanisms, in the second half of the 20th century, American and European farmers found themselves producing food in excess of need. Although some of that food was well suited to clogging up the coronary arteries, economic and educational policies were fashioned to encourage production. Sugar production and meat production became independent indices and targets of economic development, and government officials concerned with grain surpluses tailored nutritional and educational policy while under the influence of livestock and dairy producers.

The United States Department of Agriculture began to issue dietary advice to the American public in the 1890s. Then the problem was adequacy of nutrition, and there was no conflict between policies for agriculture and public health. The health problems caused by overeating had emerged by the middle of the 20th century, however, and thereafter the interests of the food industry no longer coincided with the most obvious dietary advice to maintain good health: eat less meat and fewer dairy products. Marion Nestle, chair of the Department of Nutrition and Food Studies at New York University, has traced the disproportionate influence of American food companies on a succession of recommendations and nutrition policies formulated by the United States government. In that long process, beginning shortly after World War II, the food industry has sought consistently to keep the public confused about the known relationships between food and health.[9]

In Europe there have been major differences in the development of national nutrition policies, but in my own country, the history of government nutrition policies has been broadly similar to that in the United States. The policies of the Danish government were focused on an adequate intake of calories and vitamins for most of the century, and until 1989 it had no policy concerning the relationship of food to heart disease.[10] Instead, the most influential educational materials were developed by the Danish Dairy Board ("Karolines Køkken"). They were heavily garnished with recipes requiring lots of dairy cream. That was still the case as late as 2001, in spite of years of better nutrition advice from agencies like the Danish Heart Foundation.

In 1971, I queried Erik Uhl, a senior official of the National Health Board, about the policies of the Danish government. I thought it was curious that Denmark differed so much from Norway, which had formulated policies on nutrition and heart disease as early as the 1930s.[2] Dr. Uhl told me that Denmark "most emphatically does not have a nutrition policy concerning heart disease." He said that it would simply not be acceptable to the Ministry of Agriculture.

Given the well-understood connection between coronary artery disease and the consumption of large amounts of animal products, it is salutary to consider the scale of the production of animals. There are about 1,000 million hogs in the world. A little more than 1% of them live in my country, Denmark. The 11 million Danish hogs are allowed to live for a little less than 6 months, so the annual production of hogs is about 24 million, and it is anticipated to rise in the near future. When they are slaughtered, the hogs weigh approximately 90 kg. The population of humans in Denmark is 5 million, and the weight of the average Dane is less than 90 kg. With a bit of planning, the Danish pork industry could slaughter and neatly pack the whole population of Danish humans in less than 3 months. Denmark prides itself on having one of the most efficient pork industries in the world.

Worldwide there are about 60 million horses, 57 million mules, 1,300 million cattle, 1,600 million sheep, 520 million goats, 137 million buffalos, 19 million camels, 10,000 million hens, and, as mentioned, 1,000 million hogs. The 6,000 million humans in the world eat virtually all of the pigs and quite a lot of the other domesticated animals. Much of this enormous production of animals for human food is connected to the production of cereals, and as we shall see, international authorities expect that cereal production must increase still further to meet increasing demands for livestock products.

Agriculture and the Environment

More than half of the world's farmlands are still meadows and pasture, where ruminant animals such as cattle, sheep and goats can convert pasture forage, harvested roughage or byproduct feeds, as well as non-protein nitrogen such as urea, into meat, milk and wool. One of the important developments in modern agriculture, however, has been the shift from grass to grain as feed for ruminant animals. It has contributed modestly to our rapacious use of fossil fuels, and it has contributed importantly to the erosion of top soil.

The grazing ruminant is necessary for the conversion of pasture grass to human food. In contrast, when fed on grain, which could be used directly as food for humans, the animal is an unnecessary and inefficient intermediate step along the way from synthesis of carbohydrates by photosynthesis to fuel for human metabolism. More cereals are used for feed for animals than for food for humans in the developed countries, and the developing countries are following the same path. Most of the energy content of animal feed doesn't make it through the animals to the food that humans consume: meat and dairy products contain only about 10% of the energy of the grains eaten by cattle and pigs. The rest is used by the animals for heat and locomotion.

Pasture and meadow are usually not tilled, whereas annual cultures of grain crops require tillage. Soil erosion is one, inevitable consequence of tillage. Another is that tillage requires energy, as do transportation and distribution of materials for farming and the products of farming, as well as heating, drying, etc. Other processes requiring fossil fuel may be less obvious. The most important elements of artificial, or chemical, fertilizers, are nitrogen, phosphorus and potassium. The fertilizers are produced by chemical reactions requiring energy, either because they are truly endothermic, or because they require energy to run at acceptable rates, as in the production of ammonia from hydrogen and nitrogen. The energy is obtained by burning fossil fuels, and artificial fertilizers can be considered a massive injection of energy into the production of crops.

Agriculture consumes only about 17% of the fossil fuels produced in the United States, substantially less than the 25% consumed by automobiles.[11] Nevertheless, the energy balance sheet for agriculture is dismaying. Of public concern since Frances Moore Lappé published her book on "Diet for a Small Planet" in 1971,[12] the use of fossil fuels by agriculture has been the subject of numerous studies, notably those of David Pimentel and his colleagues.[11] The dismaying part is that the way humans feed themselves is becoming increasingly inefficient at a time when overpopulation, malnutrition and soil erosion are major concerns. A shift of emphasis from the production of animals to the production of fruits, vegetables and cereals for direct human consumption would not only be healthier, it would also be more efficient, and it would reduce the pressures on arable soils and on the environment. That is not happening.

It makes little sense to blame farmers for these developments. As a result of industrialization and the dramatic expansions in the economies of developed countries, farmers had to abandon traditional techniques of production to keep their incomes competitive with other sectors of society. To get the necessary higher returns per hour of labor, they turned to large monocultures that relied heavily on fossil fuels necessary for the production of fertilizers, mechanized farming and the distribution of farm products. In the United States, more than 10 kilocalories of exosomatic (solar or fossil fuel) energy are spent per kilocalorie delivered to the customer, so that the food system consumes ten times more energy than it provides to society in food energy. In subsistence societies, on the other hand, about 4 kilocalories of exosomatic energy (mostly biomass) are required per kilocalorie of food consumed at a cost of 16 times as much human labor as in the food system of the United States.

Crop yields were beyond all expectations when the Europeans busted the sod and plowed the American prairie in the 19th century. In less than 20 years, though, yields were down to European levels. The minerals had been depleted by then, and the wind was blowing away the unprotected top soil. In this there was nothing new. Depletion of minerals and erosion of soil are unavoidable in agriculture based on tillage.[13] Nothing can compete with agriculture when it comes to destroying natural environments.

Repletion of minerals is possible under exceptional circumstances. One example is the deposition of carbon compounds and minerals during the annual flooding of the Nile valley and delta. The Blue Nile carries minerals leached from the volcanic mountains of Ethiopia, and the White Nile carries carbon compounds from the forests of Central Africa. Another example, which in a historical perspective can be considered exceptional, is chemical fertilizers in modern industrial agriculture.

Repletion of top soil is also possible, but rates of erosion are usually much greater than rates of repletion. The present Greek landscape bears witness to the erosion of ancient soils, and 90% of croplands in the United States are now losing soil above replacement rates. During the last 40 years, nearly one third of the world's arable land has been lost to erosion. Soil erosion can be checked by wind breaks, control of flooding, etc., and artificial fertilizers can supply necessary nitrogen, phosphorus and potassium, but it takes a long time to form soil with organisms able not only to facilitate the cycling of nitrogen, carbon and sulfur but also to structure the soil as a matrix for plants and other organisms. Good top soil can contain thousands of different organisms. Research to develop methods for soil formation is therefore crucial for agriculture in a sustainable form and thereby for human health in the long run.

Soil formation is not a central concern of contemporary agronomic research, however. Instead, the central concern is biotechnology. That should be changed, because top soil is more important to our future than any conceivable kind of biotechnology, however fascinating it may be in intellectual and commercial terms. One of the approaches to the regeneration of top soil is perennial poly-culture. Perennial plants live for three or more years, which gives them time to develop more extensive nets of roots. Poly-culture is the cultivation of several different plants on the same plot of ground. It is more difficult for pests and weeds to attack plants in poly-culture. Forestry employs perennial poly-culture, but industrial agriculture mostly does not. If it did, yields would go down, but top soil would be created and requirements for herbicides and pesticides would be much lower. Wes Jackson of the Land Institute in Salina, Kansas, is the most eloquent proponent of perennial poly-culture in agriculture.[13]

A doctor's prescription for a better environment would be to lower the number of livestock. The resulting lower need for grains for animal feed would drastically reduce the need to increase yields and the need for acres to be plowed. As a side-effect, it would reduce heart disease.

Agriculture and Genetics

To varying extents, all plants produce poisons to protect themselves from viruses, micro-organisms and insects. Of the millions of different plants, we use only a very small number for food, and we have either developed tolerance to the toxins in those we eat, or we know how to inactivate them when we prepare food. Anyone who has forgotten to boil certain kinds of beans before eating them will not forget the capacity of bean toxins to cause diarrhea. Mostly, though, domesticated plants contain lower concentrations of poisons than wild varieties. That might be one of the reasons for lower resistance to pests and for the resulting requirements for high-level use of pesticides. There is another and more fascinating reason, however. It is connected to the way we think about genetics, not only of plants, but also of animals, humans and human disease, and it is related to one of the great debates in biology.

"*Natura non facit saltum*" (nature makes no jumps) was a favorite dictum of Charles Darwin.[14] Like most biologists in the19th century, he was a gradualist:

> If then, animals and plants do vary, let it be ever so slightly or slowly, why should not variations or individual differences, which are in any way beneficial, be preserved and accumulated through natural selection, or the survival of the fittest?

Inherited characteristics were thought to blend or merge with each other gradually, and between a red flower and a white flower there were infinite gradations of pink flowers. That understanding of biology was called biometric, because it was based on the concept of a continuous scale of measurements.

That changed when the work of Gregor Mendel in Moravia became known in 1900, sixteen years after his death and thirty-five years after he had shown that inherited traits in garden peas could be understood in terms of discrete units of inheritance. In 1900 three other European botanists, including Hugo de Vries, independently arrived at conclusions similar to his, but on searching the literature they found his work and ensured that he was given priority for his fundamental discovery. In 1909 Wilhelm

Ludvig Johannsen suggested that Mendel's discrete units of inheritance should be called genes, but another half century would pass before the work of many scientists including Frederick Griffith, Oswald Avery, Rosalind Franklin, Maurice Wilson and finally James Watson and Francis Crick made it possible to merge the mathematical-statistical concept of the gene with a molecular understanding of the gene as a stretch of coiled DNA.

Ultimately the Mendelian school of genetics prevailed over the biometric school in agriculture and elsewhere in biology. In his book on plant resistance to pests,[15] Raoul Robinson argues that it is difficult to overestimate the importance of the outcome of this academic debate: "*The members of the Mendelian school wrought incredible damage on twentieth century crop science*". The details are complex but the gist of Robinson's argument is simple. The breeding of plants based on Mendelian concepts results in the transfer of a single desirable trait from one plant to another. The trait is usually from a wild plant to a domesticated variety, and the process is called pedigree breeding. The transfer of single genes is accomplished, not by genetic engineering, but by a form of breeding called back-crossing. In contrast, the breeding of plants based on biometric concepts results in small and gradual improvements from one generation of plants to another. It is termed population breeding, and it is due to merging and blending of the effects of many genes.

These two kinds of plant breeding result in different kinds of genetically determined resistance to pests. The resistance conferred by pedigree breeding works by only one mechanism, because it is due to the properties of one gene. In the first instance, that mechanism can be very potent, but when pests develop a way to overcome it, the plant is left with no ability of its own to resist them. Hence the dependency on pesticides. In contrast, resistance conferred by population breeding is resilient if not particularly effective against the one pest of prime concern at any one time. Some plants succumb, but most survive, even without pesticides. That's what wild plants do. Robinson argues that we could reduce the use of pesticides if the biometric principles of population breeding were more broadly applied in agriculture.

I am not a competent judge of the agronomic merits of the argument, but it rings true, and it identifies a problem in all biology. The conflict between the biometric and the Mendelian schools of genetic thinking is fundamental to the conceptual and practical problems of medicine as well as agronomy. We shall turn properly to some of the problems of medical genetics in the next chapter.

Public Concerns and the Future of World Agriculture

During the past decade, the public has become increasingly concerned with agricultural policy and especially with the evident vulnerability of our food supply. We can now, for good reasons, worry about threats of bio-terrorism, but the concern itself was primed by a lesser threat, namely the bovine spongiform encephalopathy (mad cow disease) scandal in Great Britain in the 1990s. The disease, like so many other diseases of animals, turned out to be transmissible to humans, and about 100 people died of variant Creutzfeldt-Jakob disease of the brain.[16] It had until then been rare, because it required that humans either ate the brains of other humans, as the Fore people of Papua New

Guinea once did in ritualistic cannibalism, or that brain parts were transplanted from one human to another as in corneal transplantation, a high-tech form of cannibalism. The disease is due to the tiniest infectious agents known, small proteins called prions.

The mini-epidemic of variant Creutzfeldt Jakob disease in Great Britain was caused by the transmission of prions from cows to humans. The prions were in food thought to contain small amounts of cow brain. The cows had been infected by feed containing brains of other cows. Cannibalism once removed so to speak, and a form of cannibalism that has been important especially to the European version of contemporary industrialized agriculture, because feed which has been "fortified" with animal parts contains proteins that make animals grow faster.

In 2000, the scandal widened to encompass the European continent, and thousands of infected cattle are now thought to have entered into the food chain of humans during the last two decades of the 20th century. It is not known how many Europeans have been infected, because the incubation period can be as long as 30 years. It might therefore take some time before legislation, enacted during the first years of the 21st century, will have stopped the disease. The legislation is designed to curb the use of animal parts for feeding not only cattle but also poultry and swine. This might raise the prices of food from animals, of course, and should it happen to any important extent, the legislation might change the human diet in a way that also could curb coronary artery disease (long before it has any effect on Creutzfeldt-Jakob disease). The real importance of the story of mad cow disease, however, is that it has reminded Europeans of the vulnerability of industrialized agriculture and of the precariousness of their food supply. It is also a cruel lesson in what Roy Porter calls *"the symbiosis of disease with society"*.[17]

Other societal concerns have been focused on the issues of plant biotechnology and genetically engineered food (genetically modified food). The most direct risks of the genetic engineering of food are not nutritional but, instead, the ecological effects of the transfer of genes to wild plants. In contrast, the most direct dangers to human health are the nutritional and toxicological consequences of current and future agricultural practices that are unrelated to genetic engineering. Those responsible for the administration of health care systems should therefore be aware of the projections being made for world agriculture, just as they should be aware of the projections for world health made by the World Health Organization.

Projections for Agriculture

At the end of the 20th century, the Food and Agricultural Organization (FAO) of the United Nations projected developments in world agriculture to the year 2010,[18] and the International Food Policy Research Institute (IFPRI) has made similar projections to 2020.[19] The two sets of projections are broadly consistent with each other. FAO divided the world into 7 regions closely similar to the 8 regions identified by the Global Burden of Disease Study,[20] which was also done under the auspices of the United Nations.

World-wide production of cereals for direct human consumption is expected to increase at rates only slightly higher than population growth. From 1990 to 2010, the FAO expects annual consumption to increase from 165 to 167 kg/person, with increases especially in East Asia and Latin America and some decreases in the former socialist countries. Consumption of meat is expected to increase from 32 to 37 kg/person, again with much regional variation but including an increase from 16 to 25 kg/person in all developing countries, and a very substantial increase from 20 to 40 kg/person in East Asia. That is still somewhat below the averages in developed countries, where consumption of meat will increase from 81 to 87 kg/person. Consumption of milk is expected to decrease slightly world wide, from 75 to 72 kg/person with unchanged but geographically very different patterns of consumption, probably reflecting the distribution of the gene for lactase persistence, which was discussed in the previous chapter. For example, consumption in East Asia will increase slightly from 7 to 9 kg/person, still less than 5% of milk consumption in developed countries (198 kg/person).

A 1999 report from the IFPRI extends these predictions to 2020. The IFPRI is supported by national and international agencies including FAO, the European Commission and the World Bank. The main concern of the IFPRI report is not diseases of food plenty such as coronary heart disease. Instead and more legitimately, it focuses on the greater problems of food insecurity and child malnutrition in the developing world, especially South Asia and Africa. Despite an expected decline in the number of malnourished children from 160 million in 1995 to 135 million in 2020, child malnutrition and food insecurity are expected to remain widespread. Neither food availability nor adequate health services are sufficient to combat child malnutrition, however. According to the IFPRI, as determinants of child malnutrition they are no more important than the status and education of women. It is sad that it is apparently necessary for an organization like the IFPRI to make this obvious point, which presages a theme of discussion later in this book about education and respect for complexity at the local level. Here locality is the hut, in the later discussion it will be the consultation room.

Major thrusts of the IFPRI report are the implications of the projected demography and economy of the developing countries. First, world population is expected to increase from about 5,700 million in 1995 (about 6,000 million in 2000) to about 7,500 million in 2020, and 97.5% of that increase will happen in the developing countries. Secondly, the percentage of people in developing countries living in cities will increase from 38 to 52. Third, the annual per capita income levels in developing countries will on average increase from 1,080 to 2,217 U.S. dollars but with wide variation. The increase in affluence will be particularly marked in China (from 984 to 2,873 U.S. dollars), and it will be particularly modest in Sub-Saharan Africa (from 280 to 359 U.S. dollars).

Urbanization and increased affluence affect food preference and demand. Affluence allows us to pursue culturally and genetically determined behavior patterns precluded by poverty or restricted choice. As people move from the country to the city, they eat less coarse grains like sorghum and millet, and they eat more rice and wheat. They also eat more livestock products, fruits, vegetables and processed food. The IFPRI therefore expects that demand for meat will grow much faster than the demand for cereals for direct consumption. In per capita terms, the demand for meat in developing countries will increase by 40% between 1995 and 2020, whereas it will increase by only 10% for cereals. This huge increase in production of meat is termed The Livestock Revolution. To produce so much more meat, the demand of the developing countries for feed grain is expected to increase by about 100% (doubling) to 445 million tons in absolute terms, whereas the demand for cereals for direct human consumption will increase by 40% to 1,013 million tons. By 2020, 27% of cereals will be fed to animals in developing countries, still far below levels in the developed countries, where 70% of cereals will be fed to livestock.

Based on these estimates, the IFPRI projects that the world's farmers will have to produce 40% more grain in 2020 than they did in 1995. Since most of this increase in production must come from increasing yields rather than expanding the acreage that can be farmed, the IFPRI proposes a multidisciplinary strategy to improve yields. It includes biotechnology tailored to the needs of small farmers in the developing world rather than those of industrial country agriculture, already the focus of the large life-science corporations. It also includes agro-ecological approaches with emphasis on local farm labor, organic material, improved knowledge and farm management based on farm-level research and experimentation. The IFPRI advocates an eclectic, empirical approach to exploit the biotechnology and agro-ecology that is most useful in the local setting. *"Farmers should not be made to suffer from the current debate among professionals over which approach is the most appropriate".*[19] We'll return to that discussion in Chapter 8.

Certain nutritional problems attend dependency on cereals as the major source of food energy for both man and beast. Cereals are low in protein, and they provide inadequate amounts of essential amino acids. They also do not provide certain essential fatty acids. They contain very little calcium and vitamin A, moreover, and it is difficult for the human intestine to absorb some of the other minerals and vitamins in cereals (low biological availability). Cereals are the starchy seeds of certain grasses, and to protect themselves against pests, the grasses produce substances that diminish the value of cereals for human nutrition.

Cereals are therefore not a perfect food for humans, and they were not part of our diet when our genome was formed during the hundreds of thousands of years before we became agriculturalists. On the other hand, grain is what farmers produce to feed their animals and to feed their fellow men, and without grain, human civilization would not be possible on the scale that we have known it for about ten thousand years, not to speak of the present period of a rapidly increasing world population. That is why Loren Cordain of Colorado State University calls cereals *"humanity's double-edged sword".*[21]

The degree to which we nourish ourselves by cereals varies enormously across the planet. Whereas cereals provide 17% of food energy in North America and 26% of food energy in Europe, the figures are 61% in the Near East and 67% in the Far East. That large range should be an invitation to policy makers to think about how best to balance the components of the food that is supplied to the people of their countries, and how best to co-ordinate nutritional, agricultural and environmental policies.

Ruminant animals also do not thrive on grain. In the wild, they eat fibrous plants, not grain. Like us, they do not actually produce enzymes that can break down the cellulose of plants. That is done, instead, by the micro-organisms that inhabit the rumen, the huge first part of the animal's stomach. When a ruminant animal like the cow is fed a lot of grain instead of fibrous plants such as grass, hay and beet tops, there is an overgrowth of bacteria that ferment starch and produce lactic acid.[22] The result is gaseous distension of the stomach ("feed lot bloat"). Lactic acid can also erode the lining of the stomach, and certain bacteria that thrive on lactic acid can then gain access to the blood stream and to the liver, where they cause abscesses. In 2002, Danish TV reported that, on average, 11% of bull calves had liver abscesses when they were slaughtered.

Although less than 0.3% of the cattle that are fattened in feed-lots or "factory farms" actually die because they are fed grain, erosion of the lining of the stomach must be painful, and the lives of bull calves are brief and miserable. The cattle industry uses antibiotics to reduce the occurrence of liver abscesses. Some of these antibiotics are the same as those used to treat human diseases, which is a matter of major concern to human health, because resistance to antibiotics develops much more readily. The practice of eating ruminant animals that have been raised on too much grain therefore causes diseases of animals as well as humans, and it has enormous environmental costs.

The digestive systems of pigs and ruminant animals differ importantly. The digestive system of pigs is very much like our own, and, ignoring some finer points of gastronomy, pigs eat what we eat. In Denmark, most of the grain produced by farmers is for hogs. Denmark produces about 24 million hogs each year for slaughter but less than 400,000 bull calves. In ecological terms, the pig is a bigger problem than the cow.

Global Planning for Better Nutrition

More than any other country, Finland has shown that it is possible to lower rates of coronary artery disease by public health measures. The North Karelia Project was launched in 1972 to prevent cardiovascular disease among residents of the North Karelia province of Eastern Finland. The Finnish Heart Association coordinated the initial discussions, which included community representatives, national experts, and several representatives of the WHO. Later, the program expanded to include other non-communicable diseases. The project demonstrated that high rates of heart disease can be reduced dramatically if community-based programs are planned, executed and evaluated according to clear principles and rules There must be close contact with national authorities and close collaboration with all sectors of the community, including the food industry. In the North Karelia Project, Finnish farmers agreed to increase the production of fruits and vegetables at the expense of dairy products. Berries instead of milk.[23,24]

Other countries should emulate the Finns. The WHO and the FAO of the United Nations have collaborated on plans to reduce diet-related disease (International Conference on Nutrition in Rome 1992), but the role of those plans has not been apparent in the predictions for developments in human diseases and in the developments in agriculture with which we have been concerned here. In Chapter 3 we saw that the WHO expects coronary disease to rise to the top of the list of diseases burdening the health systems of the world by 2020. The WHO report connects that prognosis to developments in smoking of tobacco but not explicitly to other developments in agriculture. Similarly, the FAO report does not explicitly connect agricultural developments to changes in patterns of human disease. The IFPRI report mentions cardiovascular disease only in passing. The whole picture of coming developments in world agriculture, however, is compatible with a general increase in food patterns associated with coronary artery disease.

It is therefore important for international agencies, especially those of the United Nations, to collaborate more extensively. Pekka Puska has been central to the North Karelia Project, and he is now director of Noncommunicable Disease Prevention and Health Promotion in the WHO. He says that such collaboration will now, in fact, happen. Beginning in early 2002, the WHO and the FAO will work towards a common agenda on diet, nutrition and chronic diseases. The two agencies, as well as other agencies of the United Nations, particularly the World Bank, are now also collaborating to find ways to curb the tobacco epidemic and to examine the potential effects, if any, that a reduction in global demand might have on various economies. The United Nations Ad Hoc Interagency Task Force on Tobacco Control, which is chaired by the WHO, has set out to study the global tobacco economy. As a member of the Task Force, the FAO, in collaboration with the WHO, the World Bank and various other UN agencies, is focusing on the small farmers of the developing countries. The FAO is particularly concerned about the consequences that a reduction in the demand for tobacco might have on the earnings and food security of farming communities that depend on tobacco harvests. Here it is being helped by the growth of populations and of income, which will expand the number of tobacco consumers across the planet. Thus, for the foreseeable future, success in international tobacco control will mean reducing the rate of growth of tobacco consumption, not causing dramatic and rapid declines from current levels of consumption. In other words, significant numbers of tobacco-related jobs will not be lost. Instead, fewer new ones will be created.[25]

In Europe, the focus of greater collaboration between government agencies is food safety, reflecting concerns about infectious diseases and genetically modified crops. According to a recent report from the European Heart Network, however, there is also some focus on more general issues of nutrition and how they are affected by a variety of European Union policies (White Paper on Food Safety in 2000, a Resolution on Health and Nutrition adopted by the Council of the European Union in 2000, and the establishment of the European Food Safety Authority in 2002).[2] It remains to be seen whether any of these promises of an integrated approach to agricultural policy and issues of human health, beyond immediate safety concerns, will be fulfilled. In its 2002 report concerning agricultural policies pursued by its member countries, the OECD (Organization for Economic Co-operation and Development) does not indicate that nutrition has been taken into account in any of these policies.[26]

How the increased consumption of meat will affect disease risk depends critically on how it is distributed within populations. Inequitable distribution of animal products could cause coronary artery disease in two ways. First, eating too many milk products and too much meat causes atherosclerosis by the well known mechanisms that I have already discussed in this book. Secondly, more recent research show that an impoverished childhood and impaired growth in the womb are associated with higher risk of cardiovascular disease later on.[27,28] Thus, poverty and poor maternal nutrition during pregnancy not only deprive children, born and unborn, of the means to grow adequately. They might also cause coronary heart disease years down the road for the child.

If more animal products were made available to everyone in developing countries, it could contribute to better nutrition in general, and it might enable women to deliver fewer stunted babies. As a corollary, it would mean that fewer people would be eating too much. Whether food will be distributed equitably is very uncertain. It is not likely to happen everywhere, for sure, and the WHO is probably right in anticipating a substantial rise in coronary heart disease. People aspiring to political office, especially in the developing world, should nevertheless make the equitable distribution of food part of their political agendas as well as election promises.

The Role of Price Structuring for Availability of Various Foods

In the previous chapter we considered genetically and culturally determined preferences for animal foods. Although they are certainly part of the problem of coronary artery disease, major economic interests in the present and coming systems of agriculture contribute as importantly to the disease. European farmers have much less access to arable land than farmers in the U.S., Canada, Australia and Argentina, and farm subsidies have therefore been especially important in Europe, ensuring that farmers have incomes comparable to those of other citizens of these industrialized countries.

Farmers grow the crops and raise the livestock that they can sell, but the market for agricultural produce tends to be strictly regulated by government. That is because of little elasticity in the demand for food. The term, *elasticity*, is a technical one that requires a bit of explanation. We all need food on a very regular basis to say the least, and that need sets food apart from most other commodities. For all commodities it is true that prices rise if buyers wish to purchase more than are available at the prevailing price. Prices fall if buyers wish to purchase less than is available at the prevailing price. Thus, there is a tendency toward an equilibrium price at which the quantity demanded is just equal to the quantity supplied. As the price rises, the quantity offered usually increases, and the willingness of consumers to buy an article normally declines, but these changes are not necessarily proportional.

The measure of the responsiveness of supply and demand to changes in price is their elasticity. Elasticity is calculated as percentage change in demand or supply divided by percentage change in price:

$$\frac{\% \text{ change in demand or supply}}{\% \text{ change in price}}$$

For example, if the price of a commodity decreases by 10%, and the sales of it consequently increase by 20%, the elasticity of demand for that commodity is said to be 2. The demand for products which can easily be replaced by others tends to be elastic, whereas the demand for a product tends to be inelastic if there are no close substitutes. In agrarian societies with huge populations, there is no substitute for agricultural produce. Food prices therefore tend to rise steeply if supply is only slightly inadequate. That's a problem for consumers. Prices also tend to fall steeply if there is more food than consumers can eat. That's a problem for farmers.

In both cases, the problems of consumers and farmers quickly become those of politicians. No politician, no king or queen, can survive for long if too many of their subjects do not get enough to eat. Marie Antoinette is a famous case in point. Politicians have also proved to be sensitive to tractors on the roads and streets, another example from France. Food prices therefore tend to be closely regulated by government, which must decide not only what farmers will be paid for their produce (price structuring), but also how much of the money collected by taxation the state will give to them either as income supports (United States) or as subsidies (Europe).

More than half of the budget of the European Union is dedicated to implementing the Common Agricultural Policy. The budget for the year 2000 was about 90,000 million euros, of which more than 40,000 million were for agriculture. In Denmark, two thirds of the total net income from farming is from European Union subsidies (4,700 of 7,000 million Danish crowns).[29]

Price structuring is most developed in Europe. The European Union buys produce from farmers at an agreed minimum price if they cannot obtain a higher price in free trade. This assurance has encouraged production of more crops than can be sold on the market. The most extreme example is the production of large amounts of wine destined not for the table but for other use including fuel. European farmers have also produced meat and butter with the sole purpose of obtaining the minimum price, and such produce has then been dumped on and disrupted markets outside of the European Union. For example, the European Union continues to produce about 6% more butter than it can consume, because the system of dairy quotas, which will continue until 2008, does not work as intended.[30] Since the world market price of butter is less than half of the price of butter within the European Union (between 3,060 and 3,460 euros/ton in 1998), the export of butter must be supported by money from European taxpayers. Almost one quarter of the 162,489 tons of butter exported from the European Union in 1998 went to Russia. Pastureland is ample in Russia, however, and Russians don't need butter from the European Union. It serves only to destabilize the market for Russian agricultural produce, because, after the dissolution of the Soviet Union, Russian farmers no longer have assurances of the sort provided to farmers of the European Union by the Common Agricultural Policy. To be sure, unstable internal markets are only a detail in the disintegration of Russian society, but that disintegration is widely perceived as threatening the economic, military and environmental security of the countries of the European Union. Nevertheless, one of the effects of the Common Agricultural Policy of the European Union might be the further destabilization of Russia. Another detail, a minor one at that, is that coronary artery disease, as we have seen in an earlier chapter, already seems to be rampant in Russia, and Russians would be well advised to avoid eating too much butter.

The problem of food surpluses in Europe has therefore been only partially solved by the MacSharry reform in 1992, followed by the Agenda 2000 reform, and Europe is gradually replacing subsidization of agricultural production with a system based on direct income supports and support for agricultural infrastructure. Direct income support for farmers makes the European system more easily comparable to that of the United States, facilitating trade negotiations between the two major agricultural powers of the world.

A period of trade liberalization was initiated with the Uruguay Round in 1991, but progress remains slow because of frank protectionism. The OECD monitors temporal changes in actual agricultural policy in the light of the principles to which member states have agreed. In its most recent report,[26] it noted that the various forms of support for farmers had been reduced since the mid-1980s, but also that there has been little recent progress in liberalization. For the time being, therefore, trade in agricultural products remains highly regulated in most OECD countries, including the United States and the countries of the European Union, and policy decisions remain major determinants of the kinds of foods that are offered to consumers.

Most consumers in affluent countries can choose the food they wish to buy and eat. They are perfectly free to choose food to promote health and to avoid food that increases the risk of disease. Virtually all public health strategies for the prevention of coronary heart disease are based on the assumption that consumers have that choice. The assumption is valid only on an individual basis, however. Indeed, it is fallacious on the population level. The reason is that animal products are exploited so efficiently by the food processing industry. The whole pig gets into human food. Parts not used or sold in time for chops and tenderloin are used in other ways. Tasty but unhealthy for all but the undernourished, they can be avoided by meticulously reading food labels. In the end, though, they will get into the stomach of someone, and it's not necessarily the cat.

The food avoided by the wise will get into the stomachs of the unwise. Each of us can choose to eat less meat and drink less milk, but as long as we, as nations, continue to produce ever increasing amounts of meat and milk, some of us will consume them, in one way or another, and on average atherosclerotic disease will continue to rise, faithfully reflecting the way we farm. The food we choose to produce determines the need for cardiologists and heart surgeons, and the choices of real importance for the health of our people are therefore not only on the level of health care policy. They are also on the level of food policy and agricultural policy.

So, it's up to us. On the one hand, Marion Nestle has depicted how the food industry, including agriculture, can influence government policies to the detriment of public health. On the other, the North Karelia Project has demonstrated that it is indeed possible to involve the food industry in a comprehensive program that has, in fact, reduced cardiovascular disease in a whole population.[9,24] The European Heart Network, an alliance of national heart foundations, has suggested a method that national governments as well as the European Union could use to work out which constellation of policies that would be most likely to reduce the occurrence of cardiovascular disease in Europe. The proposal is for an integration of agricultural, food, nutrition and economic policies.[2] Moreover, in its Agenda 2000 Reform, the European Union has begun to tie subsidization, not only to production goals, but also to environmental concerns and to small farming.[29] By modestly expanding this concept, subsidization could, on a much wider level than was the case in Finland, also be tied directly to health concerns.

Subsidies should be used to encourage

(1) cultivation and marketing of
  – cereals and legumes for direct human consumption
  – fruits and vegetables
  at the expense of meat, dairy products and tobacco.
(2) sustainable agriculture based on
  – organic farming (Europe)
  – perennial culture to regenerate top soil (North America)
  – polyculture and polygenic pest resistance in plants to lower use of pesticides
  – lower dependency on artificial fertilizers and fossil fuels

The nutritional and agricultural goals listed here are mutually consistent. The overall effect of less intensive agriculture and use of cereals for human rather than animal consumption would be

(1) health effects
  – lower incidence of coronary artery disease and associated diseases
  – possibly lower incidence of certain cancers
(2) agricultural effects
  – lower yields, more than compensated by
  – reduction of the amount of land needed for cereal production
    – lower requirements for fertilizers and pesticides
    – allocation of land for forest, pasture and recreation
  – regeneration of top soil
  – lower use of fossil fuels
  – lower production of animals
    – lower emission of animal manure and animal gases (methane, nitrous oxide, ammonia) into the environment
    – decreased use of antibiotics, hormones and heavy metals for growth promotion

The issue of producing huge numbers of animals for human food is at the core of the problems of agriculture, medicine and global food security. Increasing crop yields would, for the time being, not be necessary if

  – we could prevail upon the developing countries and the countries of Eastern Europe not to adopt the agricultural practices of the developed world, and
  – we could prevail upon the developed countries to stop feeding animals the cereals that we could eat.

To illustrate, let us make a simple calculation that ignores cereal use for purposes other than feeding animals and humans. A farmer raises cereals on 100 hectares. The yield from 70 hectares will be fed to animals and that from 30 hectares will be used directly for human food. Ninety percent of the energy in the cereals fed to the animals will be lost before it has been converted to energy in meat or dairy products for human consumption. The total food energy produced by the 100 hectares is therefore $30 + 7 = 37$ arbitrary units of energy.

By not feeding cereals to animals, the farmer could

- increase the yield of food energy from 37 to100 arbitrary units (270% increase) by raising cereals only for direct human consumption, or he could
- decrease the area used for the production of cereals from 100 to 37 hectares (63% decrease). Sixty-three hectares could then be used for other purposes including forage or pasturing of a smaller number of happier animals.

The good or evil genie of agrarian biotechnology is out of the bottle. It remains to be documented, however, that biotechnology provides better solutions to feeding the expanding human populations of the planet than the simple measure of directing some of our cereals into human rather than animal stomachs.

That simple measure would also reduce the occurrence of coronary artery disease, and it could be accomplished by modest reallocation of the vast funds in the agricultural support programs.

Corporate Farming

The OECD notes the deep structural changes taking place in agriculture. With some exceptions such as part-time farming in wealthy countries and subsistence farming in poor countries, the family farm is dying. Instead, farming has become a business, in many cases run by corporations.[26] Yet it is a concern that governments seem to have become increasingly disinclined to regulate big business.

In the United States, beginning with the Reagan administration, the federal government has accepted mergers that have created very large corporations such as Archer Daniels Midland, Cargill, IBP, ConAgra, Tyson, and Smithfield. Some of them are vertically integrated, and in many cases there is cross-ownership. The corporations are, of course, responsible to share-holders, not to voters. Politicians are responsible to voters, but money for swaying the votes comes from corporations. Apparently reluctant to use its powers to break up trusts, the American government seems increasingly less inclined to pursue agricultural policy to safeguard small farmers and small players in the food industry.[31] Quite the contrary, the Environmental Protection Agency under President George W. Bush and the Farm Bill signed by President Bush in May 2002 do little to regulate corporate farming.[32] The corporations have encouraged "factory farms," in which thousands of animals are raised in a single large building. Grain is pumped in at one end, and meat and manure come out at the other end. Such plants are called confined animal feeding operations, or CAFO's, a modern version of feed lots.

Denmark has employed factory farms for decades, especially for the production of pigs and poultry. Virtual monopolies are now also making their appearance. Several years ago the government accepted the consolidation of virtually the whole dairy industry in MD Foods. A few years later, it proceeded to accept, together with the government of Sweden, the merger of MD Foods with the Swedish dairy giant, Arla. The resulting company, also called Arla, is now the largest dairy corporation in Europe. In Denmark, it receives about 90% of milk produced by farmers. The remaining 10% is processed by a few smaller dairies, which Arla tolerates to avoid antitrust measures from the government.[33] Arla headquarters are in Viby, a small suburb south of Aarhus, just 15 minutes by bike from where I've spent most of my professional life treating patients with coronary artery disease.

The same pattern has emerged even more clearly in the pork industry, since 94% of Danish pigs are now slaughtered by Danish Crown, which is the third largest pork industry in the world. Not much smaller than Smithfield and Tyson in the United States, it is still formally a co-operative, owned by the pork farmers. In reality, it is run like any other very large business, and management did not bother to ask the farmers when it chose to buy up Steff-Houlberg, the last Danish competitor of any importance.[34] Danish Crown also sought to have a low-fat liver pâté removed from the shelves of supermarkets, because it was produced by a small, ecological competitor, Hanegal.[35] The corporation had no intention of producing a low-fat pâté on its own, but it wanted to establish its sole right to do so, even if it meant difficulties for Danish consumers in buying healthier food. The episode caused some consternation in the Danish parliament, and Danish Crown made a hasty retreat, but it was too late: everyone understood the power of the food monopolies when it came to using complicated patent legislation, not only to harass small competitors, but also to ride roughshod over health issues.

Danish Crown is the largest single pork industry in Europe. The headquarters of Danish Crown is in Randers, just a half hour's drive northward from Aarhus and the hospitals in which we work to treat patients suffering from lack of oxygen (hypoxia) to the heart muscle because of narrowing of the coronary arteries by atherosclerosis. In the late summer of 2002 another kind of oxygen deficiency could be traced to the raising of huge numbers of hogs. Lack of oxygen in the water caused the fish to swim away from the Bay of Aarhus, a beautiful part of the sea between Denmark and Sweden. The oxygen had been consumed by algae that had proliferated in huge numbers due to a combination of balmy weather and too many nutrients in the water. Nitrogen, especially, had been leached from farm fields in larger amounts than usual by heavy Spring rains. Most of the nitrogen was from hog manure and from artificial fertilizer (to raise the grain to feed the hogs). Raising hogs caused hypoxia in the sea as well as in human heart muscle.

Concluding Remarks

Coronary artery disease is just one, and not the most important, of the many unfortunate results of agriculture so dedicated to raising animals for meat and milk. Of even greater importance is that agriculture is the most environmentally destructive of all human activities, and the impact of agriculture on biological diversity and natural habitats for plants and fauna is multiplied many times by devoting so much of it to the production of animals rather than fruits, vegetables and grains for direct human consumption.

The Common Agricultural Policy of the European Union is scheduled to be reviewed in 2005, and we can hope that the consequences of agricultural policy for human health, as argued as late as in 2001 by the agricultural ministers of Denmark, Germany and

Sweden, will be included in that review. On a broader scale, it is important that the agencies of the United Nations, the WHO and the FAO in particular, develop their collaboration in order to sustain and recommend coordinated agricultural and health policies to governments around the globe.

Chapter 7

Diversity, Complexity and Human Disease

All medical students are taught the essentials of Mendelian inheritance, not only because they are at the core of our understanding of biology, but also because they explain the inheritance of many rare genetic diseases. Familial hypercholesterolemia, discussed in earlier chapters, is one of the most common of them. The evolution of molecular genetics and the merger of the statistical and the molecular concepts of the gene have only served to reinforce the legitimacy of thinking of genes and traits in exact correspondence to one another. One trait corresponds to one gene. That thinking has been further reinforced by laboratory experimentation based on cell cultures and transgenic animals in which only one or a very small number of transgenes are studied in any one series of experiments. And as if that were not enough, biotechnology and drug development can proceed quite effectively based on Mendelian concepts of genes and traits, because drugs usually have only one primary mechanism of action involving a few proteins and genes.

The problem with the popular, "Mendelian" perception of inheritance is that it provides an incomplete explanation of the genetic basis, not only of plant vulnerability to pests, but also of most human diseases. The genetic basis for most diseases of plants and animals is variation in several and often many different genes. In the realm of human disease, Mendelian concepts are of little or no help in predicting the course of a disease and the effects of intervention, which are also due to the effects of many genes interacting with each other, with proteins and with the environment. Within the context of this book, coronary artery disease, type II diabetes, high blood pressure and most forms of high blood cholesterol are diseases that are most likely due to variation in several or many genes. It is therefore not possible to understand the disease, to predict the course of the disease and to predict the outcome of various kinds of treatment, when the point of departure is concepts of inheritance based on the idea of a 1:1 relationship between genes and traits.

Gregor Mendel might have agreed. He had nothing to do with the simplifications of biology that were inspired by the rules of inheritance that he deduced from his studies of peas in the Augustinian monastary in Brünn. In fact, Mendel's "second law" of inheritance (independent assortment) of up to seven different traits at a time addressed the issue of complex genetics.

At issue here is not whether traits can be inherited as described by what has later been called Mendel's first law of heredity (the principle of segregation). That principle states that one half of the reproductive cells transmits one parental unit of heredity and that the other half transmits the other parental unit of heredity. In humans, the reproductive cells are the sperm cells and the egg cells. This principle adequately predicts how single pairs of alternative characteristics are transmitted from one generation of peas (or humans) to the next.

At issue is, instead, the readiness of the scientific and the political or industrial community to apply principles of genetics outside of their realm of validity. In this there is, unhappily, nothing new. The programs for compulsory sterilization of epileptic patients, the insane, and the mentally retarded in the 1930s were based, not only on ideas of social engineering that were typical of the 20th century, but also on ideas about population genetics for which there was incomplete or no scientific support. In her history of the Danish sterilization program, Lene Koch wrote that the leading medical proponents of the program for compulsory sterilization of the feeble-minded had not read or did not understand the calculations of the eugenic effects of such programs that had been made by the English population geneticists R. C. Punnet, Ronald Fisher and Herbert Jennings.[1] Although the geneticists were in disagreement about the exact degree to which sterilization programs could reduce the prevalence of feeble-mindedness in the population, they were all of the opinion that the effect would be very small. The sterilization programs exaggerated the importance of genes relative to environments, but, according to Koch, the Danish eugenicists felt that they were justified by the recognition that feeble-mindedness was, to whatever unknown extent and by whatever unknown mechanism, hereditary, and that the feeble-minded in any case were unfit for parenthood.

The programs were enacted in the 1930s by quite different political systems in Switzerland, Denmark, Norway, Sweden, and the United States, not to speak of Germany, and they were predicated, not only on more or less unsavory forms of social engineering, but also on an incomplete understanding of biology. The Danish eugenicists recognized that most forms of hereditary mental retardation are not monogenetic (Mendelian), but they had only vague ideas about how to handle an approach to eugenics based on quantitative and continuous distributions of genetic traits.

Perhaps it really is more difficult to understand the idea that genetic traits vary quantitatively and continuously rather than the concept of exact correspondence between gene and trait. Yet the former, not the latter, is the way biology works for the most part. In varieties of plants, in varieties of animals and humans, and in varieties of patients. We should therefore consider whether the concepts underlying contemporary programs for plant improvement and programs for unraveling the genetic basis of human diseases make sense, even in biological terms. There is a real possibility that they do not.

In this chapter I shall try to describe how our dawning recognition of genetic diversity and complexity has prepared a quandary for clinicians and biologists, and I shall try to indicate current approaches to finding ways out of it.

How Clinicians and Researchers Run Into Genetic Diversity and Complexity

Rare Genetic Variations in Clinical Medicine: Familial Hypercholesterolemia

When I came to Aarhus from Copenhagen in 1982, I was able to persuade several of my new colleagues to become interested in familial hypercholesterolemia. Over the years, we have seen many patients in the out-patient clinic of our department, and we have learned how to use molecular genetics in diagnosis and in understanding how the disease is transmitted from generation to generation in particular families. The most important thing we have learned, however, from our own experience and especially from the experience of many other physicians around the world, is that there is much more diversity than we had expected.

We have learned, first of all, that many different genetic variations can cause the same clinical picture. Initially we thought that familial hypercholestereolemia was always due to mutations in the gene for the LDL-receptor, which is the protein on the surface of cells that picks up LDL.[2] In 1987 it turned out that familial hypercholesterolemia also can be due to a mutation in the gene for apolipoprotein B, which is the protein in LDL that interacts with the receptor.[3] And in 2001, it became apparent that familial hypercholesterolemia can be due to mutations in the gene for yet another protein,[4] which is probably involved in the way the receptor works. It is naive to think that we now are at the end of the road, and we must expect that variation in the genes for still more proteins can also be involved in causing familial hypercholesterolemia.

We have also learned that hundreds of different mutations in the LDL-receptor gene can underlie the disease.[5] Each family can have its very own mutation. In quite a few families, however, we uncover genetic variations that are very unlikely to cause the protein to behave abnormally. They are innocuous rather than pathogenic. In one family we found two different mutations in the gene for the receptor that we thought might have something to do with the disease. We didn't know which one of them caused it, so we inserted the diseased gene into cells that we could study in the laboratory. If the cells received a gene with only one of the mutations, they produced LDL receptors at slightly lower rates than if they had a normal gene for the receptor. This suggested that, by itself, each one of these mutations was not enough to cause a clinical problem. But if both mutations were present in the gene, the cells could hardly produce any LDL receptor at all. So these two mutations each produced mischief only if the other was also present.[6] We don't know how they managed to do that, but the result was that they became partners in crime.

In many families with a typical clinical picture of familial hypercholesterolemia, we find no mutations at all in these various genes. That doesn't mean that there is no mutation, only that we may have been unable to find it, or that it might be in a gene we still don't know about. On the other hand, we have also learned that family members with mutations, which in other persons can be unequivocally pathogenic, can sometimes have quite normal concentrations of cholesterol in their blood.

All of this makes diagnosing familial hypercholesterolemia a challenge if we want to use molecular genetics. In many ways it is easier simply to forget about molecular genetics, because it is the patterns of high blood cholesterol and coronary artery disease in individuals and in the family that really matter, and we can treat patients quite well without knowing anything about the genes. Yet we continue to do the molecular genetics, because we are curious, and we learn so much about disease by doing them. Knowing about the genes, moreover, helps us to find other members of the family, who are at increased risk of heart disease. Most importantly, patients with familial hypercholesterolemia in general do want to understand what is going on in their family,[7] and with molecular genetic information we are better equipped to provide that understanding.

Back in the early 1980s, we thought that molecular diagnosis might be simple. Now, twenty years later, we know it isn't, and that enormous genetic and clinical diversity requires that we as molecular biologists, specially trained nurses, and clinicians must get together to discuss every new patient and every new family, comparing clinical findings with the molecular data, before we set about advising patients and families about risk of disease, treatment options and implications for children and insurance policies.

Common Genetic Variations in Clinical Medicine: apoE and Lp(a)

To get a little closer to the related subjects of diversity and complexity, let us look at a more common example of how the risk of dying (sooner than you otherwise would) can be explained by variations in two genes rather than in just one gene. Although quite simple, this and a later example from animal experimentation will give us an idea about the challenges posed by more complex systems. It also relates to the treatment of patients with coronary artery disease.

Before we do that, however, it might be helpful at this point to define what we mean by diversity and complexity. The two concepts are related, but they are not the same. *Diversity* has approximately the same meaning as variety, denoting the quality that the objects within a class differ more or less from each other. The objects themselves, however, can be simple or complex. There is diversity and variety in a box of poorly-made nails, as there is in a class of schoolchildren, but the children are more complex than the nails. *Complexity* is the quality of being intricate or complicated, consisting of many interconnected or interwoven parts. All plants and animals are complex organisms, but there is little diversity in a field of genetically identical corn, and there would be little diversity in a herd of sheep that had all been cloned from cells from the same donor animal.

In the example I want to discuss, small variations in two proteins turned out to affect how soon heart patients die and how effectively a drug postpones death. The Scandinavian Simvastatin Survival Study (4S)[8] was one of the drug trials of lowering cholesterol that I discussed in Chapter 4. In that study we had shown that treatment of patients with coronary heart disease with the drug, simvastatin, increased the chances of survival of the patients by 30% in the course of $5\frac{1}{2}$ years. It had been performed in 4,444 patients living in Denmark, Finland, Iceland, Norway and Sweden, and we had blood available for genetic studies from most of the Danish and Finnish patients. That enabled my colleague, Lars Ulrik Gerdes, to study whether genetic variation in the two proteins had affected the chances of survival.

One of the proteins is called apolipoprotein E, or apoE for short. It is a rather small protein, a string of only 299 amino acids. Virgie and Bernard Shore, a husband-and-wife team working at the Lawrence Livermore laboratories in Berkeley in California, reported their discovery of the protein in 1973. Two years later, Gerd Utermann, who was then working at Phillips University in Marburg in Germany, showed that, in humans, it commonly occurs in versions that differ from each other ever so slightly, by only one amino acid.[9] Variations of this kind are common in many proteins. Like many other proteins, moreover, apoE turned out to have multiple functions. It is, for example, involved in transporting cholesterol and other fats, not only in the blood, but also in the brain.[10] As studies of apoE were published during the following quarter of a century, many of them by Robert W. Mahley and his colleagues at the Gladstone Institute in San Francisco, the variation discovered by Gerd Utermann turned out to be very important for our understanding of the genetic background for disease.

One form of the protein increases the risk of two quite different diseases. It is called apolipoprotein E4, or just apoE4. It differs from the most common form, apoE3, by one amino acid. People who have inherited one gene for apoE4 from their father or mother are at increased risk, not only of getting coronary heart disease, but also of getting Alzheimer's disease. If they have inherited apoE4 from both their father and mother, those risks are even greater. In many respects, apoE4 works quite normally, and 15 to 20% of people in most populations have apoE4 as one or both of their two versions of the protein.

We don't really know how it increases risk of coronary disease and Alzheimer's disease. In fact, it came as quite a surprise to both neurologists and cardiologists that they suddenly found that they were studying the same small protein. It was like the last little meat ball on the dish, pierced by two forks as the light came back on in the boarding house.

The other protein is perhaps even more enigmatic than apoE. It is written "Lp(a)", and it is pronounced "LP little A". This ensures that no one outside the field has a clue to what it means. Researchers have a penchant for arcane language, and modern science is full of it. Tower of Babel.

Lp(a) was discovered in the early 1960s by Kaare Berg, who is a medical geneticist working at the University of Oslo.[11] It is a low density lipoprotein (LDL) to which is attached an extra protein that is called apo(a).[12] Recall that low density lipoproteins, like other lipoproteins, are just tiny particles of fat and cholesterol surrounded by a thin coat of protein and phospholipids (fats that contain phosphorus). Lp(a) does not appear to have any normal function. Indeed, many of us have so little of it in our blood that it can hardly be measured. So why do we have it at all?

It turns out that the gene for that extra protein, apo(a), is located on the strand of DNA at no great distance from the gene for plasminogen, which is a protein that does have important functions, because it dissolves blood clots. The two genes resemble each other, and the gene for apo(a) has probably arisen quite by chance as an imperfect duplication of the gene for plasminogen.[13] It is one of those variations that happened in the transfer of genes from parents to children. Children is the wrong word, though, because this particular genetic variation probably happened long before humans appeared on the scene. We know that, because many other animals also have Lp(a), and the European hedgehog is even able to use it for the transport of cholesterol. Therefore, if this particular duplication of the plasminogen gene happened only once in evolution, it must have happened in an animal that became ancestor to both humans and hedgehogs. For humans, Lp(a) is probably just evolutionary junk, but it can cause us trouble.

The gene and its protein come in many sizes, and when apo(a) is small, concentrations of Lp(a) in the blood are high, and vice versa. We don't know how that happens, but we know that high concentrations of Lp(a) in the blood increase the chance that some of it will get into the artery wall and contribute to atherosclerosis.

We had been interested in these two proteins for some time, so we measured Lp(a) and determined the form of apoE in the Danish and Finnish patients of the Scandinavian Simvastatin Survival Study.[14] Some of the results were what we expected. We already knew that apoE4 and high Lp(a) might increase risk, but we had not expected how much that would turn out to be the case. A patient in the placebo group was fortunate if Lp(a) was low and he had no apoE4. In that case, risk of dying before the study ended was only 6.5%. The risk was approximately doubled to 12.5% if he had either apoE4 or high Lp(a), and it was almost quadrupled to 21.3% if he had both apoE4 and high Lp(a). So genetically determined variations in these two proteins picked out patients with coronary heart disease who were at low and very high risk of dying within the next $5\frac{1}{2}$ years.

The really unexpected finding was that the drug reduced the risk of dying to the same low level (5%–7%) in all four groups. This means that those at highest risk also had the greatest benefit from treatment. In patients with both apoE4 and high Lp(a), risk was reduced from 21% to 6%. In the two groups with either apoE4 or high Lp(a), it was reduced from 12.5% to 6%. And in the group with neither apoE4 nor high Lp(a), the reduction in risk was very small, because risk without drug was only 6.5%. Treatment affected risk of a cardiovascular death, and, given the association of apoE4 to Alzheimer's disease, it is an interesting question whether treatment with a statin drug could also reduce the risk of getting Alzheimer's disease. The question is fueling a lot of research at this time, and it has not yet been satisfactorily answered.

Studies of this sort are called pharmaco-genetic studies. If they concern many genes throughout the genome, they are called pharmaco-genomic studies. Both kinds of studies tell us how genes condition the way drugs work, and the results of such studies will allow physicians to pick out the patients for whom drug treatment will be very worthwhile as well as patients for whom it is not worthwhile at all. So, should physicians ask laboratories to measure Lp(a) and determine variation in the gene for apoE, before they start patients on drugs of this sort? If our study is supported by other kinds of evidence, I think they should. Many studies of the same kind will appear within the next few years, and the era of pharmaco-genetics promises to enable physicians to tailor treatment with drugs to the genetic peculiarities of individual patients. This is a good development, because it emphasizes the relevance of taking genetic, biochemical as well as clinical diversity into account when making important medical decisions.

The figure below is an arboreal metaphor of genetic, clinical, administrative or any other kind of diversity. If we think of clinical medicine, the two first branches could be medicine and surgery, and at one of the next branchings of the medical branch we get into cardiovascular medicine. A branch or two later brings us to patients who have survived a myocardial infarction, and the substudy of the 4S trial that I have just described defines a yet finer branching into patients who did and did not have apoE4. The metaphor actually breaks down here, because it doesn't accomodate the idea of presence or absence of apoE4, each combined with high or low Lp(a). Thus it understates real diversity (several different versions of apoE) and complexity (interaction between apoE and Lp(a)). Nevertheless, it gives us a crude idea of the degree of both, because the number of branches in the metaphorical tree increases exponentially at each branch point. There are 32 branches at the fifth branching and 1,048,576 branches at the twentieth branching.

This exercise in metaphorical tree climbing should serve to suggest that we must anticipate a very large number of situations in which it would be theoretically possible to differentiate genetically between patients likely and not likely to benefit from a particular drug. It would be nice if we could, in each case, document the validity of that differentiation in a way similar to that employed in the 4S substudy. That would require an unrealistically large amount of work, however, and we shall have to develop less

Tree with normal branching.
- genetics of wild organisms

Tree with only 5 branchings
- genetics of agriculture

- clinical medicine

- managerial medicine

The number of smallest branches is an exponential function of the number of branchings:

Branchings	Smallest branches
5	32
10	1,024
15	32,768
20	1,048,576

Figure: Tree metaphors.

demanding ways of understanding clinically important genetic variability so that ultimately we will be able to tell physicians how to prescribe drugs more efficiently.

Basic scientists run into diversity and complexity as often as clinicians do, and the following example is from the laboratory rather than from the clinical wards. It provides a very simple explanation for the lack of a one-to-one relationship between a gene and the trait that happens to interest you. To belabor the arboreal metaphor still further, the next story is not about the patients on different branches and twigs. It is about how we entirely miss branch points.

Encountering Redundancy in the Laboratory

We can learn a lot about the roles genes play in physiology by adding, removing or in some other way changing the genes of experimental animals. Genes can be introduced into animals (transgenes), and genes can be removed from animals (knock-out). Examples relevant to coronary artery disease are experiments on mice that have been engineered to be without the LDL receptor on liver cells or to be without one of the proteins that bind to the receptor. The receptor picks up LDL from the blood so that it can be broken down inside the cell. ApoE is one of the proteins on lipoproteins that bind to the LDL receptor. The other is apolipoprotein B, which I discussed a few pages ago. Concentrations of cholesterol in the blood rise if the mice lack either the receptor or apoE. The cholesterol then gets into the artery walls, where it causes atherosclerosis. The experiments therefore demonstrate how changes in one gene can affect concentrations of plasma lipoproteins and the propensity to atherosclerosis.

That's not the way all experiments work out, however. In other experiments, knocking out a particular gene produces no dramatic changes in the animal. That could mean, of course, that the experiment was not designed well, and that it failed to detect the changes that knocking out the gene actually produced. But there are other possibilities. One of them is that the gene and its protein could be parts of a system of back-up mechanisms. Back-up mechanisms ensure that an important biochemical function can be performed in more than one way. Biochemical networking of this sort is likely to be present when vital functions are involved. Although it is different from the more familiar kind of biological redundancy of begetting many children, animal offspring or seeds, it serves in the same way to increase chances of survival.

An example of networking, or redundancy, in the metabolism of cholesterol became apparent in studies of cholesterol transport to the liver. They were performed by David Russell and his colleagues at the University of Texas Southwestern Medical Center in Dallas.[15] Cholesterol is a large and quite complex molecule, and, once it has been formed, it cannot be broken down again in any part of the body. Since the body constantly acquires cholesterol, however, either from food or from synthesis in various body organs, there must be robust mechanisms for getting it out of the body again. That happens mainly in the liver, which converts cholesterol to bile acids by a minor chemical modification. The bile acids then become part of the fluid called bile, which flows from the liver through the bile ducts to the small intestine, where the bile acids help to digest fat from food. that has just been eaten.

It turns out that there are several mechanisms for getting cholesterol to the liver. What was not known until recently was that in the liver there are also several mechanisms for converting cholesterol to bile acids. Again researchers used mice. They knocked out the mouse's gene for an enzyme called 7α-hydroxylase. The enzyme attaches a hydroxyl group (–OH) to the seventh carbon atom of cholesterol, the initial step in the conversion of cholesterol to bile acid. Since the knock-out mice did not have 7α-hydroxylase, they could not make bile acids, and their intestines could not absorb the fat from the chow they were given to eat. The result was skin disease and general wasting. The researchers had expected all of the mice to die, and that's what 90% of them actually did within three weeks of birth. But 10% of the mice recovered and survived normally. That was unexpected. It turned out that these survivors had a back-up system, an additional 7α-hydroxylase, the gene for which had not been knocked out. The back-up enzyme attached the hydroxyl group (–OH), not to cholesterol itself, but to a couple of so-called oxysterols, to which cholesterol is converted as part of a second pathway to the formation of bile acids. In this manner a fortunate minority of the mice had two mechanisms for converting cholesterol to bile acids. They would be the ones destined to survive in an environment full of researchers bent on knocking out the 7α-hydroxylases of unsuspecting mice.

There are other examples of redundancy in the transport of cholesterol to the liver, but this one should suffice to make the point that redundancy and biochemical networking must be expected in vital biological processes. The question in this context is what researchers do when they run into back-up systems. The data may suggest interesting biological pathways for analysis, a branch to follow, but often they just complicate matters, because sorting them out requires a lot of work.

Redundancy deserves study in its own right, however. We need to know the architecture of the tree, and David Russell's experiments showed that redundancy is not necessarily a black box, the contents of which cannot be understood. Like interactions between genes and between genes and environment, redundancy partially explains why genetic variations so often do not have the consequences we expect. One of the unfortunate consequences of contemporary emphasis on research contracts is that researchers have not been encouraged to try to figure out what is going on at branch points. They have been contractually obliged to stay on one twig only.

There is, however, increasing interest in using theories of evolution and theories of genetics in populations in order to understand puzzling data from molecular biology laboratories. For example, Diethard Tautz of the Institute of Genetics at the University of Cologne has argued that many variations in genes could have important long-term effects regarding the ability of a species of plant or animal to survive, even though they each have only extremely weak effects on the fitness of any one individual of that species. If that is true, it could go a long way in explaining why it can be so difficult to understand gene function when molecular biologists study only a few individuals.[16] Moreover, scientists are now setting up collaborative efforts to work their way through redundancy and many other kinds of biological complexity.

And now, with a few remarks about the greatest biological research project of the past quarter of a century, let us try to get an impression of current approaches to understanding diversity and complexity, especially the complexity of common diseases such as coronary artery disease.

The Human Genome Project

Easily the flagship of contemporary biology, the Human Genome Project (HGP) was formally begun in 1990 to determine the sequence of the 3 billion DNA building blocks in human DNA and to find those parts of the DNA that constitute the genes. It was mainly an American project led by Francis Collins, director of The National Human Genome Research Institute, but it had partners in Germany, Japan, France, China and especially the United Kingdom. Tasks were allotted to the participating laboratories in a manner reminiscent of the lexicographical methods used to create the great dictionaries and encyclopedias. For once, the humanities had suggested methodology to the natural sciences.

The HGP was originally planned to have worked out the sequence of the human genome by 2005, but a commercial company, Celera Genomics Group, engaged the HGP in a race to get the genomic sequence first. Ultimately the race forced Celera and the Human Genome Project into making a joint but premature announcement on June 26, 2000, that the human genome had been sequenced. The president of the United States and the prime minister of Great Britain went on television that day to congratulate both Francis Collins of the HGP and Craig Venter of Celera on the success of their efforts, which were published at the beginning of 2001. The sequence was only partial, but the HGP expects that the complete sequence will be known by April 2003.

Access to the increasingly complete maps of the genomes of plants and animals, including the human genome, is of enormous practical value for scientists. Comparisons of genomes from different species, for example, can provide valuable information about which genes are really important. These maps also contained surprises that have challenged long-held views in biology. It was expected, for example, that the human genome would contain 100,000 or more genes, but the work by the HGP and Celera indicated that it really contains only 30,000 to 40,000, not much more than the genomes of lower (less complex) animals and many plants. In fact, the true human gene tally is probably less than 30,000. That finding was a surprise for an anthropocentric science, but it illustrated that the genome could only be a small part of the whole story of biology. The differences between worms and humans could not only be in the genes as originally conceived. They had be elsewhere as well, especially in complex interactions between genes and between proteins and other components of a complex organism. Comparison of genomes of different animals have indicated, for example, that the human genome contains a larger number of expanded families of similar genes than do other genomes.

The surprise caused by the gene tally was exploited, of course, as an argument for investing more money in research into the functions of proteins (proteomics) as well as into more genomic research, but, more importantly, it brought the majority of scientists to accept what a minority had been saying for a long time, namely that animals and plants are too diverse, and biology is too complex, to be understood in terms of a simple reductionist science. That acceptance corresponds nicely with the views of most practicing physicians, who know that patients cannot be understood only in terms of the results of biochemical and other paraclinical tests. It was certainly in accordance with the views that physicians like me had developed after working for many years with the comparatively simple problems of molecular medicine.

Getting an Intellectual Handle on Diversity and Complexity

It is tempting to think that what we know about relatively rare diseases, due to a mutation in one gene, can be used, with some extra effort, to understand the much more common diseases associated with variations in many genes. The idea is almost certainly incorrect, however. In fact, Richard Strohman, who is emeritus professor of molecular and cell biology at the University of California in Berkeley, has for some time now argued that "the central dogma of molecular biology":

$$DNA \Rightarrow RNA \Rightarrow protein \Rightarrow function$$

is wrong.[17] Common diseases like cancer, atherosclerosis and type II diabetes are more complex, and they are genetic only in the fuzzy sense that many genes are involved in a complex response to something in the environment that taxes the resilience of our ancient genome. The implications of getting our thinking about these matters turned upside down are disturbing.

Type II diabetes is particularly likely to be a disease with complex genetics. The tendency to build up fat tissue probably had survival advantages in the settings of food scarcity that have been common during the millions of years of the formation of our genome, including the relatively short period since we appeared about 50,000 to 100,000 years ago as homo sapiens. Type II diabetes is rare if you use your body as intended and do not eat excessively. Since many people all over the world are doing the opposite, it is predicted that type II diabetes will have increased very substantially by 2020.[18]

Looking for Susceptibility Genes

The race is now on to find the "genetic basis" of type II diabetes, and it is safe to assume that investments in biotechnology to find a molecular-genetic solution to type II diabetes are very large indeed. Yet having that race at all is predicated on a quite remarkable assumption. The assumption is that there is something wrong with the genome in patients with that disease. That assumption is correct, however, only if it is also assumed that there is nothing wrong with the environment. That is because the disease is likely to be due to an interaction between an environment of food plenty and low demands on physical exertion on the one hand and a genetically determined excellent ability to conserve energy on the other. Most of the very common diseases with a genetic component are of this nature. At birth, only about 1% of us have a gene for a mono-genetic disease, whereas 2/3 of us are destined, sometime in our life, to get a disease that in part is due to variation in many genes.[19]

When interviewed by journalists, scientists are often quoted as saying that they are looking for the genetic cause of one of these diseases, or even that they have already found it. In reality, that's not what they are doing. What they are really doing is looking for susceptibility genes. Variation in such genes is considered to increase or decrease susceptibility to getting a particular disease. "Susceptibility to" rather than "cause of". Looking for the genetic "cause of" a disease is easier to understand, though, and it looks better on a front page or a web page.

The approach to finding susceptibility genes is to lay out signposts throughout the genome, and then to try to work out where there could be genes, variation in which increases the chances of getting the disease in question. The SNP Consortium, composed of four major laboratories of molecular genetics already involved in the Human Genome Project, was organized in the late 1990s to lay out SNP signposts in the genome. A single nucleotide polymorphism, or SNP, is the most common way by which the sequence of nucleotides in one DNA molecule varies from that in another. In the case of SNPs, or "snips" in laboratory parlance, the difference is in just one nucleotide.

If you could take a walk up or down the spiral staircase of DNA, you would encounter an SNP approximately every 1,000 steps. You wouldn't know it was an SNP unless you had taken the same walk along the DNA from the other parent or along the DNA from another person and could remember every step along the way. You've found an SNP if a particular step in the first DNA molecule is, for example, adenine-thymine, and you recall that it was either thymine-adenine, guanine-cytosine or cytosine-guanine in the DNA molecule from the other parent or another person.

If you kept walking for a very, very long time, you could make a map of where all of the SNP's are. The map can then be used to figure out which genes have the mutations that "cause" or increase susceptibility to disease. For example, if you are studying a family in which a particular, more or less hereditary, disease commonly occurs, then you would look for a pattern of SNP's that occurs only in the family members with the disease. If you are studying a group of people who are not related by family, you would look for a pattern of SNP's that occurs mainly in the people who have or who later get the disease. If the pattern occurs in the few SNP's close to or within a particular gene, then it is likely that something is amiss in that gene. You can then take a closer look at it to see whether it is in fact abnormal. The way to look more closely is to determine the sequence of all the basepairs in the gene in order to find a mutation that would change the way the gene tells the cell how to string amino acids together to make the basic structure of the protein. You would also have to work out how likely it is that the protein in question could be involved in the process by which the particular disease develops.

The idea in the SNP Consortium's discovery program was initially that identification of 2 to 3 SNPs close to or within each of the thousands of human genes would allow scientists to make the connections between gene variations and human disease and response to drug therapy. Scientists outside the SNP Consortium did not agree that this approach would work, however. Alan Templeton at Washington University in St. Louis and his colleagues studied the gene for lipoprotein lipase, an enzyme perched on the inside of blood capillaries waiting for fat to pass by so that it can pick it up, break it down and make fatty acids available for combustion in muscle or storage in fat tissue.[20] The gene that tells the cell how to make lipoprotein lipase is very susceptible to genetic variation, and some of this variation causes not only coronary heart disease but also acute pancreatitis, a painful and sometimes rapidly fatal disease. The gene is therefore a good example of the kind of gene in which we would like to be able to find variations that cause disease.

In this particular gene there is a problem that is turning up elsewhere in the genome. The problem is that variation is not evenly distributed throughout the gene. Instead, variation tends to occur in certain parts of the gene called (mutational or recombinational) hotspots. Uneven distributions of genetic variation pose a fundamental challenge to the use of only a few randomly chosen SNPs to look for variations that cause disease. Three SNPs are not enough, because too many variations will be missed. For this and other reasons, a minority of researchers felt that refinements of the approach initially adopted by the SNP Consortium's discovery program would be necessary to make a substantial number of connections between gene variation and diseases.

A refinement was discussed at a meeting in July 2001, convened by the U.S. National Human Genome Research Institute. Scientists were invited to collaborate in the construction of a map, not of common SNP's, but of common patterns of SNP's. These patterns are called haplotypes, and each of them represents a fairly long stretch of DNA. Like the approach based only on SNP's, the purpose of a map of haplotypes (the "hapmap") is to find the genes that increase susceptibility to a common hereditary disease. You look for a haplotype that occurs in patients, not in people without the disease. If the haplotype is close to, or if it actually contains a particular gene, then it is possible that something is wrong in that gene. You can then take a closer look at the gene, for example by sequencing all the basepairs. By late October 2002, the International HapMap project was underway with a financial commitment of $100,000 from government agencies in Canada, China, Japan and the United States as well as from the Wellcome Trust in London.[21]

The feasibility of finding susceptibility genes is greatest if it makes sense to look for common rather than rare genetic variations, and the scientists behind the International HapMap believe that susceptibility to common diseases could be due to commonly occurring variations in genes. Common disease, common variant. This idea is so beguilingly simple that it is already known by its acronym, CDCV. Find all the common variants and correlate them with disease. The apoE variant is in fact a very good example of a common variant that is clearly correlated to two common diseases (coronary artery disease and Alzheimer's disease), but the apoE variation might be the exception rather than the rule, and the phenomenon of "recombination" poses a major problem for scientists interested in connecting an SNP or a pattern of SNPs (haplotypes) to a susceptibility gene.

Parts of the paternal and maternal genes are shuffled, or "recombined," as they are passed on to children. The chromosome the child gets from the father also contains some chromosomal material from the mother, and vice versa. Without recombination, evolution of plants and animals would not have been possible, but recombination makes life difficult for scientists by severing the connection between a SNP, or a haplotype, and the gene that is involved in the causation of disease. In some people the connection might be there, but in others it might be absent.[22] If that problem occurs too often, it will be difficult to make the connections between the SNPs or patterns of SNPs that we know and the unknown genes we're looking for.

Some scientists believe that common diseases are not necessarily due to common variants. They believe, rather, that common diseases could also be due to rare variants. That idea is not as illogical as it might sound. Most of the variations in the human genome could be rare, but if there are many of them, they could be involved in causing diseases that appear to occur very commonly. This is one of the ideas underpinning large projects such as deCODE in Iceland, which exploits the exceptional knowledge Icelanders have about their family trees. Scientists can therefore link many small family trees of living Icelanders, suffering from certain diseases, into whole forests of stricken families.

Research teams organized by Kari Stefansson in Reykjavík have shown that comparison of DNA samples from both closely related and distantly related sufferers of a given disease enables them to identify areas of DNA that probably contain genes that are involved in causing the disease. As examples, they have found an area of the genome that seems to be linked to stroke,[23] another that seems to be linked to high blood pressure, and a third that seems to be linked to atherosclerosis of the arteries to the legs. The problem of recombination is not as great for the Icelandic researchers, because they are working with people who are related to each other by close family ties.

On the other hand, the results they obtain in Icelanders might apply to a lesser extent, or not at all, to other populations. That is because of the problem of context.

The Problem of Context

Studies of the apolipoprotein E gene can illustrate the importance of context. The protein is quite small, only 299 amino acids long. It has many different functions, and slight variations in structure, due to the replacement of only one amino acid by another amino acid, affect the risk of disease not only in the heart but also in the brain. The most important of these variations is that position 112 in most people is occupied by the amino acid, cysteine, whereas it is occupied by the amino acid, arginine, in a minority of people. The protein is called apoE3, when it has cysteine at position 112, and it is called apoE4, when it has arginine at that position. The variation is determined by the structure of the gene for apoE. The corresponding versions (alleles) of the gene are called ε3 and ε4. Roman letters for proteins, Greek letters for genes. There is nothing abnormal about having apoE4 as one or both versions of the protein (one maternal, the other paternal). In fact, apoE4 is probably the ancestral version of the protein, because it is the version that we find in the other primates. Nevertheless, as we have seen, it increases the risk of getting Alzheimers disease as well as coronary artery disease.

It is more correct to state that it increases risk only in some populations, however. In others, researchers were unable to show that apoE4 increases the risk of either coronary artery disease or Alzheimer's disease. Is that because they made a mistake, or was it because of the play of chance? Both are possible, but neither is probable, and there is a better explanation.

The apoE3/apoE4 (∈3/∈4) variation is only one of many variations in the protein and, especially, in the gene. Three other SNP's result in structural variation in the protein. The most important of them is the replacement of arginine by cysteine at amino acid position 158. The protein is called apoE2 when it has cysteine at that position, and the corresponding allele is called ∈2. A rare disturbance of the lipoproteins of blood (dysbetalipoproteinemia), which severely increases the risk of atherosclerosis, in fact occurs in people who have inherited the ∈2 allele from both parents.

Most of the other SNP's do not result in structural changes in the protein, however. They are "non-coding". A study of the apoE gene showed that people in three different populations did not necessarily have the same combinations of coding and non-coding SNP's. Although they shared some combinations, others were found only in the African-Americans, still others only in the Finns, and still others only in the non-Hispanic European-Americans.[24] Some of the combinations of SNP's, including the non-coding ones, modified the way the ∈3 and the ∈4 affected concentrations of apoE and of blood cholesterol. In other words, variations in DNA outside of the "genes" affected the way the "gene" worked.

Molecular biologists have known for a long time that stretches of DNA outside of the coding regions are involved in regulating the activity of genes. The cell uses these "regulatory sequences" to turn the genes on and off. In the case of the apoE gene, particular combinations of non-coding SNP's could be linked to particularly effective or particularly ineffective regulatory sequences that, in this case, participated in deciding the concentrations of apoE and cholesterol in the blood of African-Americans, Finns and non-Hispanic European-Americans.

These other variations outside of the coding regions of the gene are part of the genetic background for the action of the ∈4 variation, and the genetic background modifies how variation in any one gene plays out in the upper reaches of biochemistry and physiology. Even this way of looking at the variation in the apoE gene is a simplification, however. Recall, once again, that we all have two versions (alleles) of every gene, one inherited from our father and one from our mother. The two versions of the gene will often differ from each other, and there are therefore a lot of different combinations of different versions of any gene (genotypes). The theoretical number of different combinations of versions of one gene, found in a group of people, can easily exceed the number of people in the group. Typically, half of the people in a group have their own, private combination of versions of a gene. There is almost always nothing wrong with any of the combinations. They are quite normal, but they are not the same.

Had it been possible to study more genetic variations, and had it been possible to study other phenomena than concentrations of apoE and cholesterol, and had it been possible to study still other population groups, then there would almost certainly have been many other instances of complex relationships between variation in genes and variation in the way the body works and, in fact, in the way it looks. We are all human, but there are varieties of humans, some obvious, some not so obvious.

The genetic background for the effects of ∈4 varies not only within the apoE gene. It also varies in the thousands of other genes of the human genome. The potentiation of the deleterious effects of apoE on the risk of dying through variation in the gene for apo(a) is just one example. That extensive variation throughout the genome, moreover, will be slightly greater between population groups than within population groups. It is likely to be what causes the ε4 variation, and so many other variations of interest to physicians, to increase or decrease the risk of disease in one population group and not in another.

Population geneticists have been familiar with such phenomena since the beginning of the 20th century, and they have called it *epistasis*. When molecular biologists find that knocking out a gene is disastrous in one strain of mice but not in another, they are rediscovering epistasis. They use the term *modifier genes* to denote the unidentified genes that they believe have modified the effects of the gene they have knocked out. Gene modifiers are to molecular biologists what epistasis is to classical geneticists. So, even within the field of genetics, scientists with different skills use different terms to describe the same phenomenon. Tower of Babel again.

If you recall the arboreal metaphor of the previous chapter, you must now imagine that the branch supporting the patients with the ε4 variation in the apoE gene is not the outermost twig. You will have to add at least another branch point. You must imagine patients with ε4 on many different versions of the apoE gene. Each one of them is a new twig, and which one the patient happens to be sitting on could make a difference in the effects of the treatment you want to give. You must also imagine that any combination of other branches and twigs might affect the health of a patient on one of the ε4 twigs. Here the metaphor once again breaks down, because a twig on a very low branch does not normally brush against the twig of a very high branch of the same tree (unless it's a weeping willow), but that's what genes and proteins do, metaphorically speaking. They interact.

We cannot divine the terms of interaction from knowledge only of the human genome, and certainly not from knowledge only of a particular version of the human genome. What is certain, though, is that these concepts of classical genetics and evolutionary biology must ultimately be worked into the way data from molecular biology are to be interpreted, not only to further our general understanding of microbes, plants and animals, but also to make sure that we apply the results of molecular studies intelligently to the diagnosis and treatment of disease.[19]

Molecular Biology Approaches: Postgenomic Research

The data from the Human Genome Project concern all genes in the genome, not just the ones already identified and understood. The genome map is therefore a representation, albeit a simplistic one, of the panorama of human biology, and it helps scientists to find completely new areas of biology and the connections to areas already known. The SNP Consortium is only one of many large projects launched to exploit genomic data. Others are more experimental in their approach. The Alliance for Cellular Signaling, for example, is a collaboration between seven American laboratories experienced in studying how biochemical signals are received into cells and transmitted between cells. To know how such signals are coordinated, the laboratories will exploit the complete genome sequences, in a way unbiased towards particular proteins,[25] in order to characterize every protein-protein interaction in two cell types from mice and then to turn the data into a cellular wiring diagram.

Another effort, by the Institute for Systems Biology in Seattle, aims to establish how cells turn genes off and on under different conditions.[26] Beginning with the relatively simple problem of the metabolism of sugars in yeast cells, the researchers have knocked out genes, studied patterns of gene expression and measured the abundance of a large number of proteins in order to develop mathematical models of how these cells adapt to the use of one kind of sugar rather than another. Once they have built a conceptual module for sugar metabolism, they will build modules for fat metabolism and for protein metabolism, and they hope that ultimately they will be able to assemble all the modules into a complete understanding of the cell as an integrated biological system. The virtual cell.

The research to exploit the genome maps of microorganisms, plants, animals and humans has been termed "postgenomic biology". Strictly speaking, the term is a pretentious one, because it suggests that our understanding of genes and the genome is now complete. That is not the case. The gene tally generated by the Human Genome Project and by Celera, for example, is predicated on a particular concept of genes that is probably too simple. The concept is that a gene is a sequence of basepairs that tells the cell how to make one protein. A "blueprint". That is the prevalent and perhaps the most straightforward way of thinking about genes, but we know that it is not correct. I have already alluded to "regulatory sequences", which are stretches of DNA close to but outside of the coding sequences (the "blueprint"). The regulatory sequences are involved in turning genes on and off, so they are important in determining the relationship of genes to the way the body works, but they are not part of the "blueprint".

There are, moreover, several ways in which one stretch of DNA, a "gene", can make several proteins. One is by "alternative splicing", a process by which different kinds of messenger RNA can result from the same stretch of DNA. Each kind of messenger RNA will tell the cell how to make a particular kind of protein. Another is that a particular protein, once made, can be modified by the addition of various sugars or the subtraction of parts of the protein. The protein is produced in slightly different versions suitable for quite different functions ("posttranslational modification").

All this brings us back to an older concept of genes. The only one possible before the age of molecular biology, it was Gregor Mendel's and Wilhelm Ludvig Johannsen's original way of thinking about genes. I alluded to it in the chapter on the agricultural connection. According to this concept, a gene is a discrete unit of heredity rather than a particular molecule. A stretch of DNA could be a part of one gene, coding for a protein in one biochemical setting, and it could be part of another gene, coding for another protein in another biochemical setting. Thus, a gene is not necessarily one stretch of DNA. Instead, it is a particular combination of stretches of DNA, each of which can participate in combinations with other stretches of DNA to work as particular "genes" in various biochemical contexts as needs arise. Humans might be particularly good at gene jugglery of this sort, better, for example, than worms with their only slightly smaller genomes. Charles F. Sing of the University of Michigan in Ann Arbor calls this a "functional gene" concept. It is a mathematical rather than a physical concept.

The challenges to biological research, whether it is called postgenomic or not, are formidable. It is not certain that we shall ever be able to generate a perfectly coherent picture of genetic and biological diversity and complexity, and for the time being the problems described in this chapter and the preceding one remain unsolved. In recognition of this predicament, there is increasing interest in theoretical approaches to understanding complexity.

Complexity Theory

All human cultures offer religious and occult explanations of life, but attempts to work out comprehensive scientific theories of biology date back at least to Aristotle in the 4th century B.C. Attempts in the 20th century to extend the general theories of biology developed by Darwin and Mendel include catastrophe theory, chaos theory and complexity theory. The latter is the most current one, and I shall try to describe it briefly, because it helps to order thinking about complex problems in biology and medicine, and parts of it are testable. It has not, however, been developed only for biologists. It is used extensively in many other disciplines including engineering, physics, sociology and political science. Central concepts of complexity theory are irreversibility, nonlinearity, emergence, adaptation and hierarchy.[27] Let us consider each one separately.

Some of the reactions studied in physics, chemistry and biochemistry are reversible ones, e.g. the reversible reaction of carbon dioxide with water to form carbonic acid:

$$CO_2 + H_2O \rightleftharpoons H_2CO_3$$

Small boys understand that carbonation is reversible when they emit great burps of CO_2 after drinking a newly opened Coke. Some mothers seem to prefer not to understand the reversibility of carbonation.

Reversible reactions happen in the relatively simple world of the very small. In complex systems, on the other hand, processes are usually not reversible. They have direction in time. The process of ageing comes to mind without difficulty. How we lived in the womb and soon after birth, whether or not we have been afflicted with disease, how we may have eaten earlier but not necessarily now, all are likely to modify the ways genes and the immediate environment affect the risk of disease.

In complex systems, a few processes are additive (linear), but most are not. An example of a linear process is the sound wave, which can be analyzed into its component frequencies, and the whole sound wave can be reconstructed by once again adding up the components. In contrast, the processes by which an ant hill develops are non-linear. The flexibility of the ant hill in probing and exploiting its surroundings goes far beyond the total capacity of all the ants acting as individuals. The ant hill is more than the sum of its parts.[27]

The concept of emergence (of properties of the ant hill) is also central to complexity theory. It denotes a property that is impossible at a lower level but becomes possible at a higher level of a complex system. It "emerges" at the higher level of complexity. Life itself can be considered an emergent property of specifically organized physico-chemical systems: an animal is an emergent property of its cells. On a social level, I believe that coronary artery disease is an emergent property of industrialization. In all cases, something, not necessarily beneficial, has emerged from the parts, and that something is different from the sum of the parts.

Emergence of complex systems involves adaptation. An example of adaptation is the process of learning in complex biological systems. Indeed, the term "complex adaptive systems" is often used almost as a cliché, albeit a profound one derived from Darwin's theory of evolution. Plants and animals have evolved in a world shared with countless other forms of life, many of which have competed with each other for finite resources. That setting, or environment, has continuously changed, and successful species have been able to follow along, adapting themselves to, and interacting with, a world forever turning into something new.

A final invariant element of complexity theory is a hierarchy of levels of a system and of the sciences used to study them. Blaise Pascal observed that "*l'homme se trouve entre deux infinis*", because man lives in a world of things that in size are about halfway between very large structures like galaxies and very small structures like atoms. In a typical ascending hierarchy relevant to complex biological systems, John H. Holland tabulates studies of subatomic particles, overlayered by atomic physics, physics of gases and fluids to molecular chemistry and on upwards to microbiology, cellular biology, physiology and ecology (cited in reference [27]).

Somewhat closer to the subject of this book, and in a very small stretch of the range of sizes that Pascal thought about, Charles F. Sing and his colleagues have suggested a simple hierarchy. Deepest are the genes, interacting with each other and with the inter-mediate level of interacting biochemistry and physiology, and at the top is the progression of coronary artery disease as an emergent property, not only of events at the two lower levels of the hierarchy, but also of time and the environment.[28]

The central question for our present purposes is how the gene level of Sing's hierarchy is connected to coronary artery disease through the intermediate level of physiology and biochemistry. The success of gene therapy, the success of gene-based drug discovery and especially the ability to predict the course of disease and responses to drugs will depend critically on the nature of these relationships. Whether it will be possible to develop general models for connecting all relevant variation in genome to physiology and biochemistry and further on upwards to the level of clinical disease remains to be seen, however. As the 21st century opens, researchers certainly appreciate that scientific focus must shift from simple systems and few molecules to complex systems of many molecules and, once again, physiology, but a shift in the focus of interest is not the same as having a comprehensive model, and complexity theory is no substitute for a contemporary, general theory of biology.

Is a General Theory of Biology Necessary?

Richard Lewontin has argued that a new theory of biology might be unnecessary.[29] Although the concept that "genes make proteins and everything else" is certainly a gross simplification, it does not follow that we are lost without another central theory of biology, be it catastrophe theory, chaos theory or complexity theory.

> It is not new principles that we need but a willingness to accept the consequences of the fact that biological systems occupy a different region of the space of physical relations than do simpler physico-chemical systems, a region in which the objects are characterized, first, by a very great internal physical and chemical heterogeneity and, second, by a dynamic exchange between processes internal to the objects and the world outside of them. That is, organisms are internally heterogenous open systems.

If Lewontin is right, we can, perhaps, for the time being at least, muddle through without a new general theory of biology and other complex systems. It is certainly of greater immediate concern that we ignore complexity in biology and medicine than that we, for the present, cannot grasp it to the full satisfaction of our intellect. In biology we have been able to deal fairly well with diversity and complexity when we were still taxonomists and physiologists, and in clinical medicine we have dealt fairly well with diversity and complexity when clinical skill and intuition were still respectable parts of what physicians do. What is not acceptable now is the unquestioning reduction of biology to molecules and the unquestioning reduction of medicine to a few, primitive categories of disease.

Dealing "fairly well" with diversity and complexity might not be enough, of course. Richard Strohman has pointed out the problems of being "adrift in biology without a master plan", and he has argued that a general theory of biology really is necessary, and that our problem is that we don't have one:[30]

> Biogenetic engineering of humans and of plants where unanticipated results could cause damage to individuals or to millions of acres of cropland will have to cease except under tightly controlled laboratory conditions and until the time when the complexities are understood and the dangers eliminated.

Strohman acknowledges that such understanding and elimination of danger may not be possible, but he sees the present state of biology in terms of Thomas Kuhn's theory of scientific revolutions, in which a prevailing, dominant scientific world view, based on proper research and technological utility, is replaced by a contending view, a new paradigm of science.

> The structure of DNA as given by Watson and Crick was such a powerful insight about biological information, and generated such a productive wave of discovery and understanding at the molecular level, that there was every reason to believe that this information somehow extended beyond proteins to programs of behaviour. However, no genetic programs have ever been found, and here is our dilemma. We organisms are certainly "programmed" in some sense of that word, but if the program is not in our genes, then where is the program? We have no answer to this

question, and according to Kuhn, without a paradigm capable of addressing the mystery of the missing program, we will have to hang on to our incomplete paradigm of genetic determinism. Current references to nonlinear dynamics or complexity theory or chaos are all interesting starts at contributions to a new theory, but they remain as starts. That is our situation as we enter the new century. Our view of life is incomplete by half, at best.

I believe Strohman is right about the necessity of biological theory that embraces complex, dynamic systems as well as molecular genetics. Our actions are no longer only in the realm of traditional physiology and clinical medicine. We have already introduced foreign genes into plants on a very large scale, we are doing it in animals on a smaller scale, and we are doing it in humans on a very small scale. That might be alright if we knew how to prevent the transfer of such genes into other plants, especially those in the wild, and it might be alright if we really understood how genes, be they in plants, animals or humans, work in context. But we really don't at this point.

A less pessimistic view is possible, however. One of the intellectual promises, not only of genomic and proteomic research, but also of classical disciplines such as population genetics and evolutionary biology, is an elaboration of the general understanding of biology that has evolved since the beginning of the 19th century. In fact, there is a resemblance between the situation of biology then and now.

After the ecological recovery of the 18th century, European biodiversity was at its highest.[31] Romanticism was ripe, and *"Britain was full of nature. To enjoy nature, to observe, collect, classify, and arrange "natural productions" – this was a flourishing national pastime"*.[32] Naturalists were everywhere, beetling and botanizing their way through the English countryside, much like researchers in laboratories all over the world are now sequencing and snipping their way through the genomes of animals and plants as well as microbes.

Then as now, there were more data than anyone needed. They were ordered according to the 1735 *Systema Natura* of Carl Linnaeus, as some of them are now ordered by the Human Genome Project. But librarianship is not all of scholarship, and then as now there was a need for order and a way to make sense of the myriad details. Many researchers all over the world now more or less share this feeling, and indeed, for researchers it is the fundamental reason for huge collaborative research projects, some of which were briefly mentioned above.

In contrast, in the 19th century, the theory that ultimately made sense of things came out of the head of one English naturalist. Charles Darwin's was not the first theory of biological evolution, and he certainly did not work in a vacuum. Moreover, it is not unusual in science for the same idea to occur to more than one person independently and almost simultaneously, and Darwin and Alfred Russel Wallace, each drawing on his own observations in the tropics, Darwin in the Galapagos and Wallace in Indonesia, had both thought their way to a theory of natural selection by 1858.[32] It was Darwin, however, who fully elaborated the theory that remained fundamentally consistent with the later findings of classical genetics and the 20th century discoveries in molecular biology.[33] In "The Structure of Evolutionary Theory",[34] Stephen Jay Gould, building on the logic of

Darwin's original theory of natural selection, described an elaborated, contemporary theory of evolutionary biology.

Darwin had argued that selection mainly works on the level of organisms:

> Let us take the case of a wolf, which preys on various animals, securing some by craft, some by strength, and some by fleetness; and let us suppose that the fleetest prey, a deer for instance, had from any change in the country increased in numbers, or that other prey had decreased in numbers, during that season of the year when the wolf was hardest pressed for food. Under such circumstances the swiftest and slimmest wolves would have the best chance of surviving and so be preserved or selected.[33]

Gould, by contrast, argued that selection must act not only on the level of the organism, but also on several other levels from genes at the most fundamental level through cell lineages, organisms, demes, and species to clades at the highest level. Darwin's organisms are only one level of the hierarchy. Below that level are groups of cells, and futher down are the genes. At higher levels are demes (local populations of closely related plants or animals), species and clades (groups of organisms that have evolved from the same ancestor). Gould believed that selection works by different ways at each level of the hierarchy. The way genes are selected for survival differs from the way wolves are selected for survival, and, in turn, species are selected for survival by still other mechanisms including catastrophe, the mechanism that Gould expounded so well that every school child now knows how the dinosaurs died off.

Evolutionary biology is a field of lively academic controversy, and I am not competent to judge between the various points of view. Many scientists before Gould have entertained theories of biological evolution based on some form of hierarchy of the levels of natural selection, but a salient attractive feature of these theories is their kinship with complexity theory. Each level of the hierarchy can be considered an emergent property of the immediately lower level. The serious debate within evolutionary biology involves selection at the molecular level of genes[35] as well as self-organizing patterns of networks at higher levels of complexity.[36] The debate is not a theory, of course, but it is the best current discussion of a general theory of biology.

Darwin's theory and the later modifications and elaborations of the theory remain broadly consistent with what we know about biological diversity and complexity at all levels, including molecules. Indeed, as laboratory work continues to uncover ever increasing levels of molecular and cellular complexity, a Darwinian understanding has never been more relevant.

Ralph J. Greenspan has argued that data produced by basic science are much easier to interpret if we detach ourselves from the simple idea that there is one specific function for each gene and for each protein, and that a single pathway connects one protein to another. Instead, most genes and proteins are turning out to have multiple functions, and they are interconnected in multiple ways. This interconnectivity confers enormous adaptability to the cell and to the organism.[37]

> Isaac Newton might have liked the neat view of biological systems made up of dedicated components, with causal roles that can be studied in

isolation, and in which particular starting conditions give rise to uniquely predictable responses. Charles Darwin, by contrast, might have felt more at home with the idea of a complex, emergent system made up of many non-identical components, with non-exclusive roles, non-exclusive relationships, several ways of producing any given output, and a great deal of slop along the way. We have been Newtonians for the past several decades in our thinking about gene action. It is time to become Darwinians.

For sure, there are monogenetic diseases. In fact, there about 10,000 of them, but almost all of them are very rare. Each is due to the absence or malfunction of a particular gene and protein, and it is already possible to correct some of them by a specific treatment, be it with vitamins, drugs or genes, but we need still more insights from molecular biology, and we need biotechnological engagement from industry. In contrast, and as the main point of this chapter, the genetic background for the most common diseases such as type II diabetes and coronary artery is almost certainly far more complex. They are common, not because of problems in our genes, but because we live in environments quite different from the environments in which our genome evolved. It is improbable that there will ever be a vitamin, drug or gene that can correct these diseases. The idea that we can find a drug for them in biotechnology laboratories might be commercially viable, but it is likely to be scientifically naïve. Nevertheless, as we shall see in the next chapter, that is the idea on which we're basing many of our research efforts.

Chapter 8

Biotechnology and the Marriage of University and Industry

The problem with which I concluded the previous chapter can also be couched in terms that are more relevant from a business point of view. It can be summarized as follows:

Biotechnology is the application of the results of basic research in biology to practical problems in different fields including engineering and medicine. In medicine, biotechnology is eminently suited to solving problems due to the absence or malfunction of a gene or a protein that is essential for a particular biochemical pathway. Although there are about 10,000 diseases of this sort (monogenetic diseases), most of them are extremely rare. The problem is that, for many different reasons including impediments imposed by regulatory agencies, drug development takes a long time and a lot of money, and the market for a drug for a rare, "orphan" disease is often too small to justify that investment. Thus, there is little commercial incentive to use biotechnology for the purpose for which it is best suited.

In contrast, the garden varieties of diseases like type II diabetes, which are very common, are not due to the malfunction of a single gene or a single protein. Instead they are due to an environment for which our genome is not well-suited. Genomes differ slightly between people, of course, and some people have genomes that do not allow them to adapt well to a life of physical inactivity and too much food. How our body responds to that environment depends on complex and flexible networks of many genes and proteins. It may therefore be impossible for biotechnological research to result in drugs that can cure rather than merely alleviate these diseases. This is well illustrated by the history-to-date of the pharmacological treatment of type II diabetes and coronary artery disease, the success of the statin drugs notwithstanding. Yet type II diabetes, coronary artery disease and other common diseases define markets big enough to justify investments in drug development, so that pharmaceutical companies are channeling large amounts of money into biotechnology that is directed toward common diseases.

The same increasingly applies to public money. Academia has become intimately involved with biotechnology, but scientists working in universities should be concerned about all of biology, not just the part that is of interest for reasons of commerce. Academic interest in biological diversity and complexity, in basic science and in the sociological ramifications of human disease is nevertheless declining as the ties between industry and university laboratories become more intimate. Answering basic scientific questions in biology and epidemiology is becoming more difficult as the academic discipline of molecular biology merges with the applied science of biotechnology, as research becomes increasingly entangled in issues of intellectual property rights, and as closer ties between universities and industry require researchers to focus on projects with commercial potential.

To illustrate some of these generalities, let us look at what has been happening in my own country.

Biotechnology and Regional Prosperity: Medicon Valley

Between Denmark and Sweden there is a lovely strait of water called the Øresund. On the Danish side is Copenhagen, and on the Swedish side are the smaller cities of Malmö and Lund. There is now, at the beginning of the 21st century, a serious effort to fashion these three cities into a powerful transnational region of culture and industry, and politicians are asking the molecular biology laboratories of the universities of the three cities to collaborate and perhaps even merge with each other and with those of industry. The Øresund project is an example of an explicit policy of industrialization of academia that threatens interest in biodiversity and in basic science.

Further north in the Øresund is the small island of Hven. In the 16th century there was an astronomical observatory on the island, and the measurements that Tycho Brahe made there enabled Isaac Newton in the 17th century to work out the universal law of gravitation on which satellite technology is based. It illustrates the sometimes ultimate utility of basic science, now seriously threatened by emphasis on targeted and contractual research. I shall write a little more about Hven for that reason

At the center of the contemporary Øresund project is Copenhagen. This city has been the capital of Denmark for most of its history since it was founded in 1167. Until late in the 17th century it was surrounded by Danish countryside, but that changed due to a brief but ill-fated embroilment of Denmark in the Thirty Years War and to related wars with Sweden. The part of the country east of the Øresund was ceded to the Swedish crown in 1660, and suddenly the monarch in Copenhagen had nearly as good a view of Swedish as of Danish countryside when he poked his head out of the window.

Many other monarchs of Europe have had similar unpleasant experiences, but frontiers tended to be respected for several decades after long periods of European war. That was the case after the Thirty Years War, the Napoleonic Wars, and the two World Wars of the 20th century. At the turn of the century, however, 55 years after the Yalta Conference, national and regional European frontiers are once again on the move, mostly quite peacefully, as in the re-unification of Germany in 1990 and in the huge expansion of the European Union to the east that was agreed in Copenhagen in December 2002. Regions of former cultural, economic and political collaboration are also re-emerging.

In reversing the physical, economic and social decline of Copenhagen during the last half of the 20th century, the Danish government would like to recreate the 17th century region of Copenhagen and its surroundings on both sides of the Øresund as a center of commercial prosperity. Completed in the summer of 2000, the mammoth bridge across the Øresund between Copenhagen and Malmö, is one way of encouraging new prosperity. Another is biotechnology. The taxation base for Copenhagen and its suburbs could be strengthened by attracting and developing industry based on information technology and biotechnology, and the Danish government now funnels 90% of its funding for the biological sciences into biotechnology laboratories in Copenhagen.[1] In the process, it is drying up research in the smaller Danish universities. The government hopes that close collaboration between the Copenhagen laboratories and those of industry and the universities of Malmö and Lund will create a regional center to rival other European centers of biotechnology in Cambridge, Munich and Paris. The name of the new regional center is Medicon Valley, in unembarassed acknowledgement of the source of inspiration in California. The networking organization is called Medicon Valley Academy.[2]

Town and Gown in the United States and Europe

Medicon Valley Academy Ph.D. programs within the universities of the region stipulate that projects must entail "possibilities for commercial exploitation or business development", typifying the business-oriented approach to biological and other research that is pervasive at the opening of the 21st century. It also typifies the European strategic research programs, because politicians in Europe are as concerned that they have been losing the biotechnology race to the United States and Japan as the Danish politicians have been concerned about the demise of Copenhagen.

Several years ago, Barry Werth wrote an enjoyable account of the fiercely competitive relationships between a biotech company (Vertex), several major pharmaceutical companies (Merck, Glaxo, Chugai), a major university (Harvard), venture capital (J. H. Whitney & Co.) and ambitious chemists and biochemists in the development of FK 506, an immunosuppressive drug with huge market potential. European policy makers should read the book, because they should consider whether European taxation and educational polices, including university policy, really are compatible with the fiercely competitive world of biotechnology as it has emerged in Silicon Valley in California, along Route 128 near Boston, and in the research triangle of North Carolina.[3] The American faith in biotechnology has been remarkable, if faith can be measured by the money invested by venture capitalists, small investors and sometimes by universities. Investments could once pay handsomely. For example, the value of stocks in Affymetrix, the leading DNA chip company, increased more than 10 times from May 1999 to March 2000. The winners were more visible than the losers, however, and as the money turned over, most biotech companies were absorbed into others or went out of business after only a few years. In 1999 it was a rule of thumb that only 10% of American biotech firms survived as independent entities for more than 5 years.

By early summer 2000, investors had lost confidence in information technology and to some extent also in biotechnology. By the beginning of 2001, there was economic recession, which briefly deepened after the destruction of the World Trade Center in New York in September of that year. Recession then deepened further and more seriously when it became apparent that the accounting scandals in American corporations in 2002 included the very center of American political power.[4] Venture capitalism did not begin in earnest in Europe before 1999, much later than in the United States. European venture capitalists were therefore even more shaken by the recession than their more hardened American colleagues, and they were forced to write off more than three times as much of their investments in new companies in the first half of 2001 as in the first half of 2000.[5]

European universities are behind their American rivals in tying up with industry. In its year 2000 article on the new relationships of industry to universities, *The Atlantic Monthly* noted that European universities have been more aloof from business than their American counterparts. Although the latter did enjoy a long period of academic freedom after World War II,[6] American educators from Thomas Jefferson (1743–1826) to John Dewey (1859–1952) argued that universities should be engaged in the practical world. Collaboration between university and industry was especially extensive in the era of rapid American industrial growth at the end of the 19th and the beginning of the 20th century. After World War II, however, public funding assumed greater importance when the Manhattan Project and other wartime research like the discovery of penicillin and streptomycin convinced government of the ability of academics to tackle strategic research.

Public funding remained supreme until 1980, when the United States Congress passed the Bayh-Dole Act (University and Small Business Patent Procedure Act) that allowed universities to patent the results of research which had been funded by the federal government. Since then, the Congress has passed other laws to encourage ties of industry to academia including tax breaks for corporations willing to invest in university research. During the Cold War, the results of federally funded research were often closely guarded for security reasons, but the remarkable successes of Japanese business after World War II had demonstrated how industry could benefit from close ties to universities. The Bayh-Dole Act ensured that results of federally funded research could be transferred to those most able to exploit them commercially. It launched an unprecedented period of American innovation, which Europe now, somewhat late into the game, is emulating.

The economics of the marriage of university and industry are based on reciprocity and several forms of circulation of money. The expectation on the part of universities, state-owned or private, is that collaboration with industry will generate revenue directly, usually from the licensing of patents to industry, but also by university ownership of company stock. For politicians with an eye on town as well as gown, there is also an expectation of indirect earnings from increased regional prosperity and thereby an expanded tax base. Indirect earnings have turned out to be the most important by far. In 1998, more than 280,000 jobs had been created in the United States as a result of the commercial exploitation of university research.[7]

In 1999, industry accounted for about 69% (167,000 million dollars) of all investments in research and development in the United States. Most of this money was spent within industry, but 2,200 million dollars were used to fund research in universities. That may not sound like a lot, but since universities spend about 12% (29,000 million dollars) of investments in research and development, the money received from industry constitutes more than 7% of the research budgets of American universities. Money received by universities from industry can be in the form of grants with no strings attached, contracts with many strings attached, and royalties from licenses to exploit patented results of university research.

A famous example of a mix of these forms of the transfer of money is the 1998 agreement by which the Swiss pharmaceutical company, Novartis, promised to invest 25 million dollars in the Department of Plant and Microbial Biology at the University of California in Berkeley in exchange for the right to license patents held by the University of up to one third of the patentable intellectual property developed by the department. Under this agreement the university retains the patent rights, and it earns normal patent royalties from the patents. The participating faculty members, in turn, receive access to the proprietary databases held by Novartis. The Novartis/Berkeley contract is prototypical but not the most egregious of alliances between industry and university. Indeed, Robert M. Berdahl, chancellor of the University of California, Berkeley, has pointed out that many engineers have their research funded by contracts with private companies that are far more directive and protect the interests of the University far less than the Novartis agreement.

Joint public and private financing of applied research is probably more typical of Europe than of the United States, but it differs between European countries. For example, the Foundation for Strategic Research in Sweden administers public funds to support life science research performed in collaboration between Swedish industry and university laboratories all over Sweden. In Denmark, the government is concentrating its funding of biological research in the erection of the Biotech Research and Innovation Center in Copenhagen, which is to open by 2005. In BRIC, the University of Copenhagen and the Copenhagen hospitals are to collaborate with regional industry with the intention of creating a biotechnology institute, large by Danish standards and supported by grants from industry as well as government. In Germany, the Max Planck Society has entered into a multi-million dollar agreement with GlaxoSmithKline, one of the world's largest pharmaceutical companies. The idea of that joint venture, supported also by the Bavarian government, is to build a new Genetic Research Center on the campus of the Max Planck Institute of Psychiatry in Munich.[8]

Money can also flow unidirectionally from university to industry. In the 1980s and 1990s, Boston University invested 85 million dollars in Seragen, a biotech company founded by several of the university's professors. The company lost almost 150 million dollars, demonstrating that investments in the commercial exploitation of biotechnology, whether they are made by government, universities or industry, can be a risky business. As recipients of taxpayer money, government and universities should consider whether biotech companies eager to tie up with universities could be those in greatest need of university assistance. Companies with better product portfolios and research strategies could have fewer reasons to court academia.

They should also consider the overall logic of investing taxpayer money in biotechnology, because the major part of the returns on the investments must come from revenues from the sales of drugs. It is fascinating that politicians who urge investments in industrial-university biotechnology programs virtually at the same time deplore the rates of government reimbursements of high-cost drugs.

Intellectual Property

The concept of intellectual property is central to managing the research resulting from the marriage of industry and university.[9] Who owns the discovery? A commercial company wants to be assured that it can exploit the results of the research it funds, and that the results cannot be exploited by competitors. On the other hand, university researchers must publish the results of their research, not only for the sake of their academic careers, but also to maintain the mission of universities as institutions of learning and dissemination of knowledge.

Since implementation of the Bayh-Dole Act, American universities and industry have evolved an increasingly sophisticated system of patents to resolve this dilemma. The university can publish results of research, but first it must file patents that will protect the company's exclusive rights to commercial exploitation for a specified period of time. Once the discovery has been patented, the university can license the patent to industry, and the universities can retain royalties from licensing. A fraction of the royalties can, moreover, be shared as personal income to the inventors. This system has been successful. Between 1980 and 1998, the number of university patents approved annually rose from 450 to 3,200.

Many European countries have passed similar legislation only recently. The Danish government enacted law no. 347 in 1999 to encourage the patenting of discoveries made in university laboratories. The law is quite in the grain of political tradition in countries with universities under the direct control of the government. According to §7, the scientist has the right to exploit his discovery, but that right is revoked in §8, which empowers the university to take over the scientist's right if it wants to. Moreover, if there are revenues from commercial exploitation of the discovery, the university may determine how it will split the money with the scientist (§12). The law also details, at great length, the responsibilities of scientists for reporting discoveries to the university.

When Danish scientists saw law no. 347, they told the government that they would rather play golf than do more research, and the Ministry of Research responded by suggesting that revenues in practice be split with a third each to the scientist, the institute and the university.[7] That is a good deal for the scientist, and it will encourage innovative biotechnology.

The political stability of the welfare states of northern Europe make them attractive for international biotechnology companies. There is a problem, however. The confiscatory taxation underlying welfare can deter biotechnology companies from moving operations to Denmark and similar countries. It can also encourage talented researchers to move to countries with advanced biotechnology and lower taxes, for example the United Kingdom and the United States. The governments know this, and they have been reluctant to abandon principles of economic equality between citizens in favor of more lenient taxation that will permit scientists to make 10 times as much money developing drugs as school teachers make teaching children to read. That is not a trivial dilemma.

Partnerships, if not marriage, between industry and university is less problematical in engineering than it is in biology. Inventions are truly made in schools of engineering, but discoveries rather than inventions are usually made in biology. Taking out patents on such discoveries has caused profound unease, only slightly relieved by the subtle and perhaps sophist requirement that it is the adaptation of life processes to industry rather than the life processes themselves that can be patented.

There is also little comfort in public rather than private ownership of patents on life processes. State-owned biotechnology laboratories, erected to serve the state itself in a contemporary quest for riches, are not really different from the expeditions financed by the kings of Portugal and Spain in the 16th century. The captains of those expeditions also claimed discoveries, geographical ones then, for Christianity, but especially for their most Christian and Catholic majesties, and researchers, politicians and industrialists would undoubtedly like to believe that the biotechnology race is about basic research as well as about pharmaceuticals. The emphasis, though, is on the discovery of genes, proteins and simple biochemical pathways that can be exploited for applied pharmaceutical research. The emphasis is neither on disinterested, basic research, nor on applied research into the myriad specific and local forms of complex biology.

Basic Science

The former Danish minister of research said of the Biotech Research and Innovation Center to be built in Copenhagen: *"The distance between basic research and its applicability has become much shorter, and that necessitates more integrated structures"*.[10] The integrated structures she envisaged as minister are almost certain to violate anything that can truthfully be called basic science.

Let us consider, therefore, a bit of basic science by returning for a moment to Renaissance Denmark and to the Øresund, now the northern part, which surrounds the little island of Hven. Tycho Brahe was a young law student at the University of Copenhagen when a total eclipse of the sun in 1560 kindled a life-long study of astronomy. His measurements showed him that existing tables of planetary movements were inaccurate, and he decided to devote his nights to the movements of heavenly bodies, or at least to the measurements thereof, while he studied jurisprudence during the day.

In 1573 he published his discovery of a new star in the constellation of Cassiopeia. Since stars were supposed to be perfect and unchanging, the discovery of a new star was inappropriate, and it further undermined the Aristotelian views of the universe. His work was not on the revolutionary scale of that of Nicolaus Copernicus in Poland, but it established his European reputation, and it was recognized by King Frederik II. In 1576 the king gave Tycho Brahe title to Hven, now a favorite destination for summer outings by ferry and sailboat. The king also gave Brahe the means to build an astronomical observatory, and Brahe's meticulous astronomical measurements on Hven later enabled Johannes Kepler in Prague to work out how the planets orbit the sun. Especially Kepler's third law, which related a planet's mean distance from the Sun to the time it took the planet to orbit the Sun (1629), was essential for Isaac Newton's work in Cambridge.

In 1687 Newton published the foundation of modern physical science, Principia Mathematica, in which he formulated the universal law of gravitation: every particle of matter in the universe attracts every other particle with a force that is proportional to the product of their masses and inversely proportional to the square of the distance between their centers. If engineers did not know that, they could not calculate orbits for space satellites or trajectories for space travel. What is certain is that Frederik II had no inkling of the consequences of giving the island of Hven to Tycho Brahe. He did not care that Brahe's research was not immediately useful. He only wanted his little kingdom to be part of the excitement that later became known in Europe as the *Dawn of the Enlightenment.*

Horizons are limited, especially in democracies, where terms of political office are short. Persuading politicians to make long-term investments in research can therefore be difficult. In 1971, Julius H. Comroe Jr, director of the Cardiovascular Research Institute of the University of California in San Francisco, gave it a try. He noted that basic research in American laboratories had begun to suffer due to budgetary restraints, conscious preference for goal-directed research and the use of research contracts rather than research grants. Those developments have only accelerated since then, but Comroe's counter-arguments are still valid. He argued that the nature of the discovery of new treatments, the value of which are not disputed, must be understood if universities are not to be destroyed.[11]

He offered examples. The newspapers had concentrated on only the surgery when writing about the transplantation of the human heart as one of the dramatic achievements of 20th century medicine. But what the readers, and the politicians, really should have known about cardiac transplantation was all that went on before the surgeon began his work. To make a long list short: use of the stethoscope, the electrocardiograph, cardiac catheterization, x-rays, angiocardiography, pulmonary function tests, and more.

> Does Congress know how each of these diagnostic tests or instruments came into being? Was Roentgen, in discovering x-rays, looking for a way to study the heart? Was Einthoven, in discovering the string galvanometer, searching for a way to diagnose arrhythmias? Was Werner Forsmann, in performing the first cardiac catheterization, looking for a way to measure left ventricular end-diastolic pressure?

Comroe didn't really need to continue, but he did. Who was responsible for the development of the science of immunology? How was anesthesia discovered? Who discovered asepsis? Who discovered bacteria? Who discovered antibiotics? And who discovered positive pressure ventilation without which the chest could not be opened?

The science policies now being pursued, including the pervasive use of contractual research goals, ignore the way most important discoveries are made, be they astronomical or medical. It is ironic that applied research is now displacing basic research and simultaneously capitalizing on the promises that only basic research can fulfill.

When Comroe wrote his essay, student rebellions on the other side of the Bay of San Francisco at the Berkeley campus of the University of California were in fresh memory, and he concluded his essay by exhorting "*us not (to) put ourselves in the position of the militant students who want to destroy universities without having something better to offer"*. Thirty years later, it is clear that the threat to the universities came not from the students. Quite the reverse. In 1964 students at Berkeley had criticized the university for bending over backwards *"to serve the need of American industry"*, and in 2000, it was again the Students for Responsible Research at Berkeley that criticized the Novartis deal as being *"in direct conflict with our mission as a public university"*.[6]

The Danish Minister of Research was told almost the same thing in 1997, when Jens Christian Skou of the University of Aarhus in Denmark received half of the Noble Prize in Chemistry for his discovery forty years earlier of the enzyme in cell membranes that pumps sodium out of the cell and potassium into the cell. If it were not for that pumping action, nerves could not transmit impulses to muscles, and muscles could not contract. Indeed, animals with nerves and muscles would not have been possible, and Skou told the Minister of Research that his work would not have been possible under the current system of contractual research. The Minister listened politely, but only six years later, in 2003, the reform of the university system proposed by her Research Commission will make it possible for industry to exercise unprecedented influence on the universities. I shall return to that proposal in just a few paragraphs.

Academia Forever Balanced Between Isolation and Engagement

In his indictment of the direction of modern science, the American essayist, Wendell Berry, wrote this:

> The patron (becomes) the prescriber of the work to be done. (Patronage) removes the scientist from the human and ecological circumstances in which the work will have its effect, and which should provide one of the standards by which the work is to be judged; the scientist is thus isolated, by this principle of following patronage, in a career with a budget. What this has to do with the vaunted aim of pursuing truth cannot be determined until one knows where the money comes from and what the donor expects. The donor will determine what truth (and how much) will be pursued, and how far, and to what extent.[12]

The politically anointed marriage of university to industry endangers not only the university's commitment to basic research. It also endangers the universities as institutions of critical thinking and real education.[6] But there are two sides to this coin, for once an appropriate metaphor. One side is that commerce and war can be powerful instigators of science, and academia can turn stale behind closed doors to the university. The European explorations of the 15th and 16th centuries, however motivated by greed for gold and conquests, ultimately did provide a much more coherent and correct picture of our planet. And in the 19th century, the purpose of the voyage of the HMS Beagle to South America and the Galápagos was to survey the oceans so that imperial Britain could control them better for commerce and war. The purpose was certainly not to allow a passenger on board, Charles Darwin, to make the observations necessary for a theory of biological evolution. During World War II, Alan Turing played a leading role in decoding secret German naval messages. That work led him to work out the principles for a computing machine that foreshadowed the development of digital computing.

The other side of the coin is that closed doors and ivory towers are also necessary. Darwin made his observations during the voyage of the Beagle, but he did not announce his theory until 27 years later. In the meantime, he did a lot of thinking in Down House in the green hills of Kent. Gregor Mendel worked out the theory of discrete inheritance in the quiet gardens and the library of the monastery in Bruno, and Alan Turing was, if anything, a quiet, reclusive thinker. The origins of molecular biology and biotechnology are therefore certainly to be found in engagements in commerce and war, but also in reclusion and prolonged hard thinking. It seems, therefore, that universities must forever balance themselves, as well as they can, between engagement and isolation.

Tipping the Scales

The immediate future of many important universities is increasing engagement in commerce. In Denmark, the universities are all funded by the state. There are three real universities in Copenhagen, Aarhus and Odense, and there are eight schools of pharmacy, engineering, etc., which have recently been elevated in status to "universities". By late 2002, the work of the Research Commission had resulted in a proposal for a new law regulating the structure of all of these universities. Until 1970, the "konsistorium", or governing body of the university, had been elected by the professors, but as a result of student revolts in the late 1960s, it was thereafter elected by and composed of junior as well as senior academics, technical personnel and, since 1973, of students. Democratization lowered the competence and authority of the konsistoria and of the faculties of the university, and it entailed a complicated electoral process and a cumbersome bureaucracy, but the universities remained fairly autonomous. That will now change. The law to be passed by the Danish parliament in the Spring of 2003 will replace the konsistorium by a board of directors, the majority of whom will be people from outside the university, perhaps from industry.[13]

Restructuring the universities will make them better suited to collaborate with and train young people for industry. The race is on to find the "genetic basis" of high blood pressure, high blood cholesterol and type II diabetes, but these common diseases are "genetically based" only in a limited sense that happens to suggest a biotechnological solution. Biotechnology will speed up drug development, and drugs help patients who already have disease. Some drugs, moreover, are really quite good antidotes to the worst of the food that we eat. For better or worse, they will come from goal-oriented research of small biotech companies and large pharmaceutical companies working closely with universities almost everywhere across the globe.

Nevertheless, changing the way we live our lives as city dwellers would be a more efficient way to prevent diseases like type II diabetes and coronary artery disease. Those of us with enough knowledge, determination and money can do that on our own, but most of us will continue to suffer from maladaptation to urbanization unless we adopt more enlightened policies for health care, schools, city planning, and agriculture. These complex economic, social and political issues are far more important than problems that can be solved by any form of biotechnology. They are less sexy, and they are less commercially remunerative for private and public investors. To the extent that they are predicated on academic understanding, however, these issues should be the objects of critical inquiry in university faculties of economics, politics, sociology and agronomy that are not controlled by business people. And to the extent that we need to know more about the relationship of the environment to lipids, sugar and countless other biochemical components of blood, we shall need new approaches to complex biology and ecology that can only come from disinterested, basic research in universities that are not forced to take commercial potential into consideration.

A similar but not identical conclusion pertains to agriculture. Daniel Charles has written a balanced history of recent agricultural biotechnology, particularly the story of transgenic, or genetically modified (GM), crops.[14] At the center of the story are the researchers in the agrochemical company, Monsanto. Early on they saw in bio-technology, quite idealistically, the possibility to create a new, clean agriculture. The traditional form of industrial agriculture depended heavily on the massive use of pesticides, which had become the focus of fierce popular and political opposition inspired by Rachel Carson's "Silent Spring" (1962). In 1980 the U.S. Supreme Court cleared the decks for biotechnology in agriculture as well as in medicine. It ruled that living organisms, created in the laboratory, could be patented, and companies like Genentech, near Stanford University in California, surged ahead in human biology. In agriculture, companies also worked closely with universities. In collaboration with Washington University in St. Louis, for example, Monsanto launched a research program to develop GM plants. Similar efforts got underway in Europe, where the pharmaceutical company Hoechst worked closely with the University of Bielefeld in Germany.

After much effort, Monsanto and Hoechst as well as smaller companies (Plant Genetics Systems in Belgium) succeeded in introducing genes into plants that made them resistant to the herbicides that already were being sold by the companies (Roundup and Basta). The advent of herbicide-resistant crops was not the clean technology originally envisaged, however. "*It brought biotechnology and pesticides to the marriage altar in a fateful embrace*", but it was certainly biotech in part, and it became a source of huge revenue, especially for Monsanto.

In contrast, the development of plants containing the Bt. gene was unadulterated biotechnology. The microbe Bacillus thuringiensis secretes a protein that is deadly to several caterpillars that can destroy crops. Monsanto and the University of Washington in St. Louis, in sharp competition with other universities and companies, including Ciba-Geigy and Plant Genetics Systems, worked out a way to get the gene for the fatal protein into corn, tobacco and cotton. The protein was harmless to humans but deadly to certain caterpillars, and concern arose in 1999 that it might also kill the larvae of the Monarch butterfly when they fed on the leaves of Bt corn. The Monarch butterfly therefore briefly became a beautiful symbol of nature vulnerable to the side-effects of agricultural biotechnology, but by the end of 2001, further research had shown that little damage was done to desirable insects such as the butterfly. In a commentary on that research, David Pimentel and Peter Raven of Cornell University in Ithaca NY wrote that, compared to the damage wrought on ecosystems by destruction of habitats and by the widespread use of pesticides, Bt corn could actually have huge benefits for the survival of many species of insects including the Monarch butterfly.[15]

In the mid-1990s, Monsanto began to buy up American seed companies, and by 1998 it was the world's second-largest seed company. It expected a large market for gene-modified crops, but in the course of the 1990s, popular opposition to gene-modified grains and soy beans had developed, especially in Europe. The European Union did not actually disapprove of GM crops, and it did not actually prohibit the import of grains that had been genetically engineered, but the governments of member states were reluctant to approve GM crops. Moreover, major European processors of food, such as Marks & Spencer and later Nestle and Unilever, were sensitive to popular concern, speculative and emotional as it might be. There emerged a de facto European boycot with substantial implications. "*Europe had become a fortress against the expansion of genetic engineering*", wrote Daniel Charles, and the huge American processor of grain, Archer Daniels Midland, decided, for example, that GM crops were not worth the effort. There was no economically feasible way of transporting huge amounts of corn and soy beans in such a way that genetically engineered varieties could be kept apart from non-engineered varieties destined for European consumption.

The International Food Policy Research Institute has argued that, appropriately used, biotechnology could become an important element in feeding the ever increasing populations of city-dwellers, especially those in the developing countries.[16] In the developing world, though, there was also less interest in GM crops than expected. The reason was also economic, but it was not the same as the reason that caused Archer Daniels Midland to renounce genetically engineered grains. Most farmers in the developing countries quite simply could not afford to buy the new seeds. Charles points out that farmers in the developing countries are not farmers in the North American (or European) sense of the word. They are just poor residents living in rural villages, and they have no money to buy Monsanto's seeds. "*If biotechnology offers any benefits for such farmers, those benefits will have to emerge from non-profit institutions or from the relatively ill-equipped facilities of publicly funded laboratories in the developing world*".

The use of genetically modified crops did increase very rapidly from 1996 to 1999, but since then it has leveled off. GM soybean in Argentina now occupies more than 90% of the national soybean area and GM cotton more than 70% of the cotton area in the U.S. However, of the total global area (conventional and transgenic) of the 271 million hectares given over to the planting of soybean, canola, cotton and corn in 2000, only 16%, the equivalent of 44.2 million hectares, were planted with transgenic varieties. Moreover, these 44.2 million hectares were very unevenly distributed across the planet. Almost all them were in the Western Hemisphere. In 2000, the United States raised 68%, Argentina raised 23%, and Canada raised 7% of transgenic crops.[17] China grew 1%, and European farmers grew virtually none.

By the end of the 1990s, Monsanto was over-extended by the purchase of seed companies, the market for genetically engineered crops had deteriorated, and the value of the company's stocks had fallen. In December 1999 Monsanto merged with and briefly became a subsidiary of the Swedish pharmaceutical company, Pharmacia, itself now engulfed by Pfizer.

Life Sciences

Although I have tried to draw attention to similarities between biotechnology of agriculture and medicine, I must also stress one of the less obvious differences. In agriculture, farmers already raise crops that are genetically identical, not because of contemporary biotechnology, but because of traditional forms of plant breeding (pedigree breeding). Opposition to agricultural biotechnology is therefore, at least in part, speculative (Europe) or economic (developing countries), and it is not primarily rooted in the intrinsic problems of biological complexity. In medicine, on the other hand, biotechnology based on current, simple concepts of how genes determine biochemical and physiological processes, does not allow us to understand the most common and most economically burdensome diseases such as coronary artery disease and type II diabetes. In contrast to the crops that farmers raise, patients with these diseases are genetically all slightly different from each other. It is for different reasons, therefore, that the major problems of human disease and the major problems of the production of food may not be amenable to solutions from biotechnology.

That being said, the progress of biotechnology in agriculture and in medicine seems, for the time being, to have arrived at a common destination, which is the production of drugs. The future of GM crops being uncertain, the immediate future of plant biotechnology may lie in pharmacology rather than agriculture proper. Appropriate selection of plants and genes for transfer into plants can make them produce drugs. That activity is, accurately, called "pharming".

This is an important and to some readers, perhaps, a less than acceptable conclusion. It is hardly surprising, however. The links between the pharmaceutical and agricultural industry have been close for a long time. For example, in the 1970s, several pharmaceutical companies began to buy up seed companies (Pfizer, Ciba-Geigy, Sandoz and Upjohn), and in the early 1980s, some of them set up laboratories to work on plants (Pfizer, Hoffmann-La Roche), just like Monsanto was also doing. Pharmacia, a pharmaceutical company, briefly engulfed Monsanto, before Pharmacia itself was bought by Pfizer. Aventis is the result of a union of the agricultural operations of Hoechst (AgrEvo) and the French pharmaceutical company, Rhone-Poulenc. Common laboratory methodology supports the dual interest in the biology of plants and humans, which has been subsumed under the concept of "life sciences".

If, then, the biotechnology of agriculture and the biotechnology of medicine are emerging as primarily of interest to the pharmaceutical industry, and if biotechnology at the very best can provide only partial solutions to the problems of adequate nutrition and adequate health care, is it not irresponsible to dedicate our universities to that particular branch of the applied sciences? We could question whether applied sciences really belong to a university. If we do accept applied sciences as one branch of university research, we should at least insist that there are other branches of science in a true university. A tree with only one branch is not a tree. Basic natural science and critical sociological, economic and political science are at least as important. As we have seen, however, developments taking place in Danish universities, and in all likelihood in many other universities subjected to the same pressures across the planet, are likely to relegate these disciplines to areas of secondary interest.

Within biology, David Ehrenfeld of Rutgers University in New Jersey argued several years ago that whole branches of science such as comparative biochemistry, comparative physiology, taxonomy, marine invertebrates, mammology, ornithology, biogeography and limnology are being forgotten at American universities.[18] And *The Atlantic Monthly* wrote that less commercially oriented areas of science languish as university-industry ties grow more intimate.[6] Universities everywhere have thrown themselves into a race to position themselves as advantageously as possible in the ranking of centers for biotechnology.

The idea that biotechnology will provide simple solutions to the complex problems of agriculture and human health is, perhaps, more prevalent in the United States than it is in Europe, where we have been more willing to confront the economic, social, political and ecological complexities of agriculture.[14] Nevertheless, Medicon Valley and other European attempts to emulate American biotechnology show that, on both sides of the Atlantic, there are researchers, politicians and business people who, for the simplest pecuniary reasons, are willing to sacrifice the independence of the universities and the diversity of university research. If, as seems depressingly possible at this juncture, biotechnology continues to fail to deliver real solutions to the major problems of medicine and agriculture, we shall have little use for universities that have been reduced to doing biotechnological research and training students for careers in the biotech industry.

We shall then be without the universities that could have performed dispassionate inquiry into myriad problems including the deeper and more complex causes of human disease and the ills of agriculture.

Chapter 9

Medicalization

Busy physicians cannot always take the larger biological, sociological, historical or political view of the ultimate causes of any particular disease, however germane they might be to fundamental forms of prevention. They must take care of patients who are ill. Dealing with the ultimate causes of the illness can come a little later, perhaps never. Treatment is imperative, whereas prevention is facultative. This pertains not least to heart disease. Patients with heart disease are often acutely ill, and diagnosing and treating acute disease has been and remains a large part of cardiology and cardiac surgery. Prevention must come a little later. A job for someone else, perhaps.

Within the limits to be discussed, the historical disinclination of physicians to deal with prevention has nevertheless changed during the last decade. That is because of an important development in medicine including the disciplines of cardiology and cardiac surgery. It is the gradual perfection of acceptable forms of human experimentation, especially the randomized clinical trial, and the emergence of a system of beliefs that we call evidence-based medicine, which depends on the randomized clinical trial, over a much longer period of time, more than fifty years. Much of evidence-based cardiology concerns preventive measures such as drugs to lower cholesterol, diet and even the smoking of tobacco, and this documentation has in fact caused physicians, including cardiologists and cardiovascular surgeons, to take a broader view of the diseases they treat. That view now includes a range of preventive strategies such as stopping smoking, lowering blood pressure and cholesterol, inhibiting the coagulation of blood, and using drugs like ACE-inhibitors to prevent deterioration of the structure of the heart muscle. The broader view of coronary artery disease is not infinite, however. It continues to be quite strictly limited to what is considered testable by the method of the randomized clinical trial, which is at the core of the concept of evidence-based medicine.

It is also limited by the recovery of biological determinism after a few decades of revulsion at the atrocities committed by Japan and Germany in the 1930s and 1940s. At the beginning of the 21st century, the idea has again become paramount that genes determine proteins and everything else. Furthermore, this time around, there is no legitimate form of socialism to challenge biological determinism in individual and social life. Confidence in our ability to fashion the world to become a better place in which to live was undermined as the failures of socialism became progressively better known at the end of the 20th century. Some of the most obvious failures to protect the environment were in fact in the socialist countries, founded on assumptions that included the idea that the people's state would be able to assure its people of the most responsible exploitation of natural resources. That irony and many others were lost on no one, and stocks in political ideology founded on social theory are at the beginning of the 21st century at an all time low.

At the confluence of biological determinism and loss of confidence in our political institutions to plan our future wisely, it is possible to find fertile ground for the belief that medicine rather than politics must provide relief for countless ills, aches and worries. Medicalization is a special case of reductionism, because it reduces problems to those that can be solved by drugs and surgery. It is an important part of the larger history of medicine in the 20th century,[1] and this chapter is therefore quite focused on how we think about pharmacological and surgical solutions to the problem of coronary artery disease.

I shall first attempt to indicate how I think some patients think about it. As we become ill, we become thoughtful. Disease, or fear of disease, makes you think about what causes it and what it can do to you and perhaps your family. Patients with coronary artery disease know that they are using drugs and subjecting themselves to surgery for a disease brought upon them by life in an increasingly man-made and artificial world. It is a world quite different from the agrarian world of our recent ancestors, and it is even more different from the world of the hunter-gatherer and his predecessors, which formed our genome and which is still imprinted in our minds after thousands of years of agricultural civilization. Those patients who fish or hunt or gather mushrooms for fun know a little about that.

I shall then try to indicate what physicians like me think we know about treating and preventing disease. Increasingly we believe that the randomized clinical trial tells us what we need to know to help our patients best. In fact it often does, but it has assumed such pre-eminence that it has eclipsed other sources of medical knowledge, and it has deflected our attention from those clinical research questions that it cannot address. For better or worse, it is also one of the most important links between physicians and industry.

And in the next and final chapter, I shall attempt to describe some of the problems that have attended the adoption by managers of the health care systems of the methods of clinical epidemiology, including the randomized clinical trial.

Medicalization and Patient Perceptions

We all have a sense of the dualism of artifact and nature. Many of us do not mind mixing art and nature, but others are more finicky about the dualism, and it is pertinent to the way patients look upon drugs as a way of life. Here are two stories about this.

Walter is a construction engineer. His work is mostly at his desk or in his car, and he loves what he calls good food. At the age of 45 he is only slightly overweight, and he is cheery and unconcerned. His wife is not. She knows that Walter's father died of a heart attack just before his 50th birthday, and she persuades Walter to see a physician about his own risk of a similar death. Although he doesn't smoke, his blood pressure and blood cholesterol have both, on several occasions, been on the high side.

His physician recommends a Mediterranean version of good food as well as weight loss to the level Walter had when he was 25 years old. Walter tries to lose weight, but with little success, and after 3 months of mostly ineffectual attempts to change his "lifestyle", Walter begins drug treatment to lower his blood pressure and blood cholesterol. He feels perfectly fine about this turn of events, and it bothers him not in the least to take medicine, probably for the rest of his life. Good drugs to accompany good food.

Walter has a cousin. Her name is Betty. She has just passed 50, slim and trim, and she looks younger than Walter. She is worried about heart disease and especially about osteoporosis. She drinks herbal teas and abhors drugs, but she can't figure out what to do about milk. She consults physicians fairly frequently, and they do not agree on milk. One tells her to drink a pint a day to protect her bones. Another says it will raise her cholesterol, and she thinks of her father's brother, who was Walter's father, usually more than Walter does. She really would like to drink more milk, though, because it seems to her a more natural way to ensure life-long healthy bones than taking calcium tablets. In the overall scheme of things it doesn't make sense that a "natural" food that protects her bones at the same time can endanger her heart.

The overall scheme of things was not part of my training in medical school, and the discussion takes more time than suits my hospital administrator. A waste of time, he thinks. Nevertheless, this is what I said to Betty:

Heart disease and osteoporosis are both irrelevant to any sensible overall scheme of things. Ability to escape heart disease and osteoporosis has had no obvious survival advantage for our ancestors, because if they got them at all, they got those diseases long after they had finished raising their children. Many of our genes, in all other respects compatible with good health, and many of the environments down the path of our evolution, might well have been conducive to osteoporosis and heart disease. It was of no consequence. Milk doesn't really protect us against osteoporosis, but even if it did, it is unlikely to have been the mechanism by which it helped some of our ancestors to survive. Milk does contribute to heart disease, but that is unlikely to have lessened its survival advantage.

The reasons that milk increased chances of survival are obvious. Milk is a good source of fat, protein and carbohydrates, produced by animals eating grasses that humans cannot eat. But part and parcel of being a milk drinker is that you can use the animals for other purposes as well. They provide good manure, and some of them can pull your plows and wagons. When they've done that, you can kill them for meat, horns, hides, leather and soap.

So I told Betty that whoever worked out the overall scheme of things probably doesn't care that the milk she thinks is building her bones could also clog her coronaries. She listened carefully to my tale of the scheme of things as I saw it, manure and everything. Then she said she already knew all that, and that she still didn't want to take calcium tablets.

"Then drink skimmed milk," I said.

"I already do," she said. "A pint a day."

The hospital administrator is right, I thought.

Most physicians have first-hand experience with these and many other differences in patient attitudes to drugs, especially those used for preventive purposes like calcium tablets or drugs to lower blood pressure. Physicians themselves can also have quite different opinions about the matter. In the consultation room, it can be difficult to withhold drugs that demonstrably lower the patient's risk of coronary artery disease. In any larger setting it makes less sense than a social and political one, but physicians should not be blamed for using drugs to counteract the effects on susceptible patients of an environment they each can only influence in small ways. The question is where to draw the line about susceptibility. At what level of susceptibility should drugs be used? We cannot resort to cardiovascular drugs and surgery on an epidemic scale without implicitly rejecting the idea that there are perfectly rational political decisions to be made to curtail the epidemic of coronary artery disease.

There are deeper political reasons for concern about a medical solution to problems that are fundamentally social and political. Betty would subscribe to a point of view advanced by Francis Fukuyama in a recent book about biotechnology.[2] Fukuyama argues that our current use of neuropharmacology indicates how we might exploit the even greater potential of biotechnology. Antidepressive drugs like Prozac, and psychoanaleptic drugs like Ritalin, are widely used for purposes in addition to those for which they were first developed. Prozac is indicated for clear-cut mental depression, but it is increasingly used to treat slightly depressed women lacking in self-esteem ("self-esteem in a bottle"). In child psychiatry, Ritalin is indicated for serious attention-deficit-hyperactivity-disorder, but it is increasingly used to help normal children, boys especially, to sit still in class. Tom Sawyer was clearly a case of Ritalin deficiency.

Fukuyama notes that using drugs for existential and social problems erodes our sense of human nature and human dignity. There is little dignity when self-esteem and acceptable behavior depend on the ability to buy drugs rather than the ability to cope with a bit of adversity and misfortune, but there is also a more important implication. Our political institutions (in democracies) are based on a code of human rights and a sense of human nature, and, however difficult to define, the latter, human nature, must be traceable to our biology. The rub is that human biology, by definition, is changed by drugs as it will be changed, more fundamentally, by manipulation of our genes. We cannot change our own way of thinking, as we already do on a wide scale with current neurotropic drugs, and we cannot entertain the idea of enhancing intelligence or physical prowess by genetic manipulation, without eroding our shared ideas of human nature. The erosion can happen without the manipulation of the human genome on a wide scale. Acceptance of the propriety of genetic modification to create humans with enhanced abilities is implicitly a rejection of the idea of an inviolable human nature on which modern democracies are based.

Fukuyama shares this concern with many others. Several years ago, Roy Porter wrote that *"with transplant surgery established and human cloning feasible, modern biomedicine is seriously challenging and changing our notions of what a human being is, of what it is to be human"*,[1] and Leon R. Kass noted more recently that *"science essentially endangers society by endangering the supremacy of its ruling beliefs"* (as cited in reference [3]). In the old days, all men were created equal and endowed with certain unalienable rights. That can now be fixed by biotech.

Evidence-based Medicine

At the core of the system of beliefs that we call evidence-based medicine is the randomized clinical trial. Like molecular biology and biotechnology, it is merely scientific method, but after many years of honing, it has now been almost perfected, and it is the pre-eminent source of information to guide physicians in making clinical decisions. Before discussing the problems that I believe result from that pre-eminence, a few paragraphs about the method and the system of beliefs.

If a drug always alleviates pain, cures a rash or takes away the fever, within hours or days, there is not much doubt that it works. Physicians like to prescribe, and patients like to take such drugs, especially if there are few or no side-effects. But most drugs are not like that. Some might seem to relieve pain, but a placebo tablet, which contains no active drug, turns out to work as well or almost as well.

Other drugs relieve no pain, cure no rash, and they do not lower temperature. Instead they are intended to reduce the risk of suffering another bout of the disease or the risk of getting the disease at all. If a drug of this kind has no side-effects, you might not even know that the tablets you are taking contain any active drug. You are taking them on faith in the evidence that your physician says is there or which you see is there by reading a bit of the literature easily accessible in book stores, libraries and on the internet. The term, evidence-based medicine,[4] is almost an incantation, but it denotes a real advance in identifying the basis for rational selection of diagnostic methods or forms of treatment. It is the integration of the physician's own clinical experience with the best available scientific evidence.

In the classical hierarchy of evidence, the least important include the results of basic research, because they have usually been obtained in test tubes, in cells or in animals. Somewhat better are observations of patients who, for some reason or another, have or have not been exposed to some form of treatment. The best evidence is from randomized clinical trials and from meta-analyses of such trials.

The statin trials of lowering cholesterol, discussed in earlier chapters, are good examples of randomized clinical trials that demonstrated, to everyone's satisfaction, the benefits of a treatment which until then had been considered controversial. The patients who had been chosen at random to be treated with statins for five years lived longer than the patients who had been chosen at random to be treated with placebo tablets for the same time period. In contrast, other trials have shown that treatments, widely used on the assumption of benefit, do not in fact work as expected. The story of hormone replacement therapy of women after the menopause is one of the most recent of several good examples. Many women, American women especially, have taken estrogens after the menopause to protect themselves from heart disease. They have done that because their physicians have been impressed by observational studies showing that women who happen to be taking estrogens also happen to have lower rates of heart disease. The problem is that associations of this sort do not establish causality. Women who take estrogens are also wealthier than women who do not take estrogens, they eat better food, they are physically more active, and they do not smoke as much. Nevertheless, for most physicians it came as a surprise when two large trials of hormone replacement therapy failed to show the anticipated reduction in coronary artery disease.[5–7]

Other cardiovascular trials have shown that other kinds of treatments clearly don't work. Several kinds of drugs combat abnormal heart beats, which can be bothersome as well as dangerous. One of the most effective classes of such drugs is called class I antiarrhythmic agents. The classification is based on the manner by which the drugs affect the electric impulse that passes through the heart to make it contract and relax. Cardiologists and non-specialist physicians therefore used these drugs quite extensively until 1989, when the *New England Journal of Medicine* published the preliminary results of a randomized clinical trial. Two of these drugs, flecainide and encainide, had been tested for their ability to reduce death rates in patients who had survived a myocardial infarction. The expectation was, of course, that the drugs would improve survival because they were effective in combating some of the most dangerous kinds of abnormal heart beats (ventricular arrhythmias). But the expectation was dashed. When the codes were broken, it turned out that death had claimed more patients in the group treated with active drugs than in the group treated with placebo. Later confirmed by the results of two other trials, the publication of the Cardiac Arrhythmia Suppression Trial[8] chastened the practice of cardiology and accelerated the search for better drugs and other ways of treating the most serious irregularities of heart beat.

Another beautiful theory to be killed by a nasty fact is the antioxidant story. Basic research had shown that vitamin C, vitamin E, beta-carotene and several other substances could prevent the oxidation of LDL, which is known to contribute to atherosclerosis. That fitted nicely with epidemiological research showing that eating food with a large content of antioxidant vitamins appeared to reduce the risk of coronary artery disease. There were many prominent proponents of the antioxidant idea. During the last years of his life, Linus Pauling, a double Nobel Prize laureate, argued that vitamin C especially, would protect against disease. The makers of vitamin tablets, and huge numbers of commercial outlets and stores profited from the story, but it began to unravel with the publication of properly performed clinical trials, and the largest of them, the Heart Protection Study, showed that simple supplementation of the diet with vitamin tablets provides no protection from coronary artery disease.[9]

The statin trials, the estrogen trials, the antiarrhythmia trials and the vitamin trials belong to an increasing number of trials with clear-cut implications for clinical medicine. Thousands of cardiovascular trials have been performed, and hundreds are underway with thousands of patients. There is now good evidence of benefit for a long list of treatments to prevent or to lessen the symptoms of heart disease.[10] They include drugs that lower blood pressure or cholesterol, drugs that inhibit the clotting of blood by a variety of mechanisms, drugs that prevent irregularities of heart rhythm and drugs that cause the kidneys to produce more urine. If capsules of fish oil are considered drugs, they should also be on this list. With somewhat greater difficulty, randomized clinical trials have also been used to test surgical procedures. Angina pectoris can be effectively relieved by coronary by-pass surgery or by dilatation of the coronary arteries by catheters passed through the large arteries from the groin. In acutely ill patients, these procedures probably also prolong life.

Where possible, medical therapy should therefore be based on the results of randomized clinical trial. When such trials are well designed and well executed, one or two of them can resolve long-standing contentious issues and create the consensus among physicians that must precede major improvements in treatment for many patients. Smaller trials can also be very useful, if a properly performed meta-analysis of many such trials produces a clear result. One of the purposes of The Cochrane Collaboration is to produce such meta-analyses (http://www.cochrane.org). The Cochrane Collaboration is so called, because from the early 1970s to his death in 1988, Archie Cochrane, a British epidemiologist, had drawn the attention of physicians to the need for systematic, continuously updated reviews of clinical research evidence. At the close of the 20th century, this international collaborative effort had been partially successful, but representatives of the Cochrane Collaboration have sometimes been attacked when they call attention to the low quality of the evidence justifying some forms of therapy and diagnosis.

Randomized clinical trials have had profound effects on the practice and administration of medicine, and evidence-based medicine is virtually identical with the philosophy of modern clinical medicine. It is also central to the policies pursued by the pharmaceutical industry and by health care management. Nevertheless, there are important limitations to the concept of evidence-based medicine.

One of the most important is that many problems of clinical medicine simply do not need to be resolved by the results of randomized clinical trials. Treatments that have immediate and obvious benefit, such as setting a bone fracture, stopping a bleeding and giving insulin to a patient in diabetic coma, need no randomized clinical trial to test them.

Another limitation is that most of the problems of clinical medicine pertain to patients who cannot be included in randomized clinical trials. Virtually all of the approximately 10,000 monogenetic diseases are each so rare, for example, that it is impossible to test the value of any particular treatment by the usual version of the randomized clinical trial. Countless other problems of clinical medicine cannot be or have not been addressed by the randomized clinical trial. There have been no recent, major outbreaks of anthrax, but should a bioterrorist unleash one, we shall have to treat victims based on what we know from animal experiments rather than trials performed in humans.[11]

More importantly, testing hypotheses by the randomized clinical trial is easier, quicker and cheaper if the patients entered into the trial do not differ too much from each other. The more variation between patients, the more difficult it is to identify a true difference between drug and placebo. When we fall ill, most of us are not textbook cases, however, and many of us who might want to be included will in fact be excluded from trials because of one or two of a host of sources of clinical variation (too old, too young, wrong sex, presence of another disease, drinks too much, doesn't smoke enough, doesn't like doctors, likely to move, etc.).

If clinical variation is a problem for inclusion into trials, it is an even greater problem when it comes to interpreting the results of the trial. For obvious reasons, everyone agrees that the results might not pertain to the patients who, for one reason or another, were excluded from participation. Physicians must treat all patients, however, and they must therefore "extrapolate" the trial results to patients who could not have been included. Extrapolation is based on a whole series of untestable assumptions, but it is a necessary exercise in daily clinical practice.

In contrast, it is often assumed that the trial result at the very least must apply to all patients who could have been included in the trial. That assumption is not correct, however. On average, patients in the experimental group might have done better than patients in the placebo group, but they did not benefit equally. There would have been little variation in the result if they had all benefited equally, but there is always variation. When we analyze the results of large trials, it is always possible to identify subgroups that appear to have benefited more or to have benefited less than the average patient. Some of this variation is due to the play of chance, but at other times it reflects real differences between patients. In Chapter 7, I described a substudy of the Scandinavian Simvastatin Survival Study which showed that benefits of treatment were much greater in patients who had a particular variation in the gene for apolipoprotein E. I believe that this is an example of real differences between patients. Although other studies should be done to test that particular idea, there can be no doubt that there is important variation between patients, and that the overall result of any particular trial only applies with certainty to the "average patient."

The "average patient", however, does not exist. He or she is a mathematical abstraction. The implication is that a physician, even when practicing medicine based on results of randomized clinical trials, cannot avoid clinical judgment. Even if his patient would have fulfilled inclusion criteria, there is no way of knowing that he or she in fact will benefit from the treatment that the trial showed was beneficial to the theoretical "average patient". Physicians must therefore diagnose and treat their patients on the basis, not only of the results of clinical trials, but also on the basis of their experience and their knowledge of anatomy, physiology, biochemistry, etc.

The reason that this is so is inherent in the method of the clinical trial, which, like all the other methods of clinical epidemiology, is stochastic. It is based on laws of probabilities. The randomized clinical trial is nothing but an experiment on humans, performed as stringently as possible within limits necessary to protect participating patients from harm. It is done to test whether a form of treatment, which observational studies of human populations or animal experiments suggest is beneficial, in fact turns out to be better or worse than placebo. When the result is known for the non-existing average patient, however, the decision to treat or not to treat a real patient must depend on clinical judgment. The idea that clinical decisions can be reduced to searching the evidence from randomized clinical trials is therefore quite untenable, despite what we might say as clinical scientists, department directors and managers of health-care systems. It is a form of reductionism that compromises clinical medicine just like molecular reductionism compromises biology.

Medical Technology Assessment

A completely different kind of limitation to the concept of evidence-based medicine is that we can disagree about the extent to which medicine as practiced should be required or allowed to be based on the evidence. We might say "evidence-based medicine", but what we sometimes mean is "medicine based on the evidence we agree to like". Let me provide examples first and generalize later.

The major part of health care in all countries, including the United States, is financed by "*more or less compulsory levies on the general population, within or outside the formal tax system*".[12] Reimbursement of expenditures for drugs is a sizeable chunk of health care and understandably the object of administrative and political scrutiny. The evidence that cholesterol-lowering drugs, on average, safely lower risk of death by coronary artery disease had been established by meta-analysis in 1994, and from 1994 to 2002 it was further substantiated, ad absurdum, by the statin trials. I described a bit of that history in an earlier chapter. The Danish health authorities, citing economic reasons, have nevertheless continued the policy of limited reimbursement that it had pursued since 1977. That policy changed, but only a little, when two colleagues and I did a simple calculation for the benefit of the newspapers. Prominently published, it showed that government policy caused one death per day in Denmark. The policy was then relaxed but not to the level of reimbursement applicable, for example, to the sulfonylurea group of drugs, which are used to treat patients with diabetes.

Whereas injections of insulin are used to lower blood sugar in patients with type I diabetes, oral drugs are usually used to lower blood sugar in patients with type II diabetes, which is a more common condition. The evidence underpinning the pharmacological lowering of blood sugar in patients with type II diabetes is very limited, however, and we really don't know whether the sulfonylurea drugs, especially, do the patients any good. Nevertheless, the use of these drugs is deeply entrenched in clinical practice, and many physicians have felt that it would be unethical to test this kind of treatment in a clinical trial. For that reason, not only have very few trials been performed in patients with diabetes, but the design of the best and most recent of them was so complicated that it left several important questions unanswered.[13] The poor state of the evidence for drug treatment of patients with type II diabetes is now considered one of our biggest challenges in clinical medicine.

Ignoring evidence is not limited to medicine. In many countries, psychologists have tried to help people recover from a traumatic event of some kind. In most cases, "psychological debriefing" to prevent post-traumatic stress disorder is voluntary, but some institutions have made it compulsory in order to reduce the threat of litigation. It has in any case been very popular, originally with the military, but later also with civilian organizations including hospitals, banks, police, railroad companies, and the Red Cross, the employees and customers of which can be victims of countless forms of extremely unpleasant experience. A Cochrane review of 11 randomized studies of psychological debriefing nevertheless failed to turn up any evidence that did any good. The trend was the reverse, and the conclusion was that "*compulsory debriefing of victims of trauma should cease*".[14] Organizations are nevertheless likely to continue to use psychological debriefing, not only for litigational reasons, but also because it is a relatively inexpensive way to do something for people in evident distress.[15] Better to do something wrong than nothing at all.

Thus, the idea of evidence-based medicine, and evidence-based health care, can at times be pitted against strong political and cultural forces. Under ideal circumstances, the evidence turned out by clinical trials is subjected to a systematic process of review called medical technology assessment, which also takes into account important economic, organizational and political forces. During that orderly process, administrators and politicians will sometimes decide against implementation of a treatment that is well supported by the scientific evidence. That is as it should be, although one might personally disagree with that policy, as I did in the issue concerning reimbursement of the cholesterol-lowering drugs. Quite often though, as indicated by the examples just given, the process is less orderly, and special interests prevail.

Evidence-based Medicine and the Relationship of Clinical Medicine to Industry

The pharmaceutical industry might well be seen as the prime instigator of the medicalization of society, but that view is too simple. Roy Porter writes, correctly, that *"modern medicine has become synonymous with complex infrastructures and towering superstructures: with universities and professional organizations, multi-national pharmaceutical companies and insurance combines, hospitals doubling as medical schools, research sites and lobbies, government departments, international agencies and corporate finance"*.[1] The whole complex, not just the pharmaceutical industry, depends on the idea that there are medical solutions to the countless problems of modern life, and evidence-based medicine has emerged as one of the principal justifications for the participation of academic and orthodox clinical medicine in medicalization.

As originally described, evidence-based medicine was a sensible but somewhat inflexible set of guidelines for making rational clinical decisions,[4] but with time it has been elevated to doctrine, and it is now used for purposes that are quite different from meeting the lowly needs of physicians in charge of patients. It is used for marketing purposes by the pharmaceutical industry, for administrative purposes by managers of health care systems, and for litigational purposes by lawyers prosecuting physicians for negligence.[16] In short, it has become integral to the workings of the Leviathan of modern medicine. I shall discuss management and litigation in the next chapter, and I'll conclude this chapter with a few remarks about the connections between clinical medicine and the pharmaceutical industry.

We have an impressive catalogue of invasive and non-invasive diagnostics, of ways to relieve symptoms of stable coronary disease, ways to manage acute coronary disease with drugs and surgery, and ways to prevent recurrence of disease by drugs and individual counseling about diet and smoking. The catalogue reflects the enormous investment into clinical research during the past 60 years, and it is what gathers tens of thousands of physicians and other interested parties at the gargantuan annual meetings of the American Heart Association, the American College of Cardiology, and the European Society of Cardiology, to name just the largest of them.

Anyone experienced in attending these meetings will know that you must arrive at hot-line sessions 15 minutes before they are supposed to begin. All the seats have been taken five minutes before the session, and people are sitting on the floors of the aisles at 1 minute to start. Two minutes after start, ponderous men force their way through doorways past tiny hostesses trying in vain to enforce the regulations of the local fire department. Why all the commotion? It is because most of the hot-line sessions are devoted to presentations of results of the latest randomized clinical trials of drug treatment or of instrumental diagnosis and therapy. Of the 18 hot-line presentations at the 22nd Congress of the European Society of Cardiology in Amsterdam in August 2000, sixteen were presentations of drug trial data, and the remaining two were epidemiological surveys with direct bearing on the use of drugs. The presentations are therefore of keen interest to the marketing departments of pharmaceutical and instrument companies. It is a lot safer to be a hostess at the sessions for basic research.

Most of randomized clinical trials are funded by the pharmaceutical companies. The research budgets of the companies can be very large, and a tiny fraction of it has in fact supported my own close work with Merck, Bayer, Eli Lilly, Squibb, Astra, Parke-Davis, Schering-Plough and Pfizer on randomized clinical trials. Some of that work has resulted in data that have become useful in clinical practice, and I have obtained support from the companies for research into areas in which they could have only moderate if any interest. With one exception, all of the trials in which I have participated were initiated by clinicians who persuaded the companies to invest money in a trial to test an idea that we, the clinicians, had thought up. Despite such close ties, I believe that the research policies pursued by drug companies, like those of medical societies and government, must be understood and discussed, because they profoundly affect health care, whether it is delivered by private or government hospitals.

In the research laboratories of several pharmaceutical companies, marketing people work closely with scientists, even during a drug's early development, to ensure that there is an appropriately large market for any drug the scientists are developing. Some of the larger companies reckon that annual revenues during the patent period should be about one billion dollars to justify the development of a drug that can be expected to meet the substantial requirements of the Food and Drug Administration in the United States.

Calculations of market potential are legitimate, and they are necessary for all stages of drug development. The problem is not primarily the obvious self-interest of industry. The problem is the deflection of interest from a huge number of largely unfundable clinical research questions to those in which industry has a more obvious interest. Too often, therefore, the questions addressed are interesting mainly from the point of view of marketing. In scientific terms, they can be less interesting, and at times they are trivial. They do not always deserve the investments that are ultimately made by physicians working in public hospitals, and they deflect physician interest from questions of non-drug and non-instrumental therapy, research concerning small groups of patients, virtually without market potential ("orphan diseases"), and basic epidemiology and biology. The deflection of interest to questions more relevant for pharmaceutical and instrumental industry parallels exactly the withdrawal from basic to applied laboratory research that we discussed in the chapter on the marriage of industry and university.

Thus, despite tremendous recent increase in our understanding of diseases such as coronary artery disease, at least three phenomena in the world of medicine and surgery, two of which have become important during the past half century, make it difficult to appreciate the cultural context in which coronary artery disease occurs, as well as the social and political links in the chain of events that cause coronary heart disease. The first is that diagnosis and treatment must always take precedence over prevention. Treatment is imperative whereas prevention is optional. The second is the re-emergence of a simple biological determinism that has replaced sociological inquiry diminished by the apparent failures of social ideology in the 20th century. The third is, paradoxically to some readers, the emergence of evidence-based medicine. Although of inestimable value to clinical science, the generation of trial evidence and the implementation of the results of clinical trials consume economic and intellectual resources at the expense of answering other research questions and at the expense of studies of the political, societal and agricultural context of diseases such as coronary artery disease.

Chapter 10

Managing Medicine

The way of life in advanced market economies and now also in the developing world produces large flows of patients with coronary artery disease. Although the flows are constantly changing, as indicated by the results of the MONICA Project, the changes are now also thought to be at least partly predictable, as illustrated in the Global Burden of Disease Study. Moreover, treatment of patients with coronary artery disease, as currently practiced in advanced market economies, is expensive, and one of the concerns of the World Heart Federation is how that challenge of costs will be met by developing countries.

The combination of disability, loss of life, large numbers, perceived predictability, and high costs makes coronary heart disease one of the diseases of major interest to health care planners. It appears to be well suited to cost monitoring and quality control efforts, two of the main responsibilities of hospital management. In this last chapter I shall discuss the managerial context in which patients with coronary artery disease are now being treated. I will attempt to show that practical problems that invalidate current attempts to control the quality of diagnostics and treatment are so well known that they are textbook material. More importantly, I shall try to argue that the fundamental assumptions of current attempts to control quality of treatment are flawed, and that attention to the diversity of clinical medicine as a result is suffering in the same manner as attention to diversity is suffering in science and in agriculture.

Management of Health Care

Caring for the sick is now called "health care". It is a Newspeak term, but I shall use it, uncomfortably, in the following.

The primary responsibility of the management of hospital systems is to deliver "health care" of acceptable quality to patients at acceptable costs. Around 1970 it became apparent to Americans that costs were accelerating unacceptably. That realization came 5–10 years later in the other OECD countries, where costs were not increasing as rapidly as in the United States. The Organization for Economic Cooperation and Development comprises the industrialized, market-economy countries. In percentage of gross national products, average health expenditures increased from about 4% in 1960 to slightly more than 8% in 1993 in OECD countries. In the United States, expenditures increased from slightly more than 5% to more than 14% in the same period, whereas in the United Kingdom, costs did not reach the 1964 levels of American expenditures until 1981.[1]

Controlling costs required larger bureaucracies. Again bureaucracy increased to a greater extent in the United States than in other OECD countries, in part because the political failure in 1994 to reach agreement on a comprehensive reform of the American health care system allowed numerous different health care plans to proliferate across the country. Bureaucracy has increased in the health care systems of all countries, however, not only to control costs, but also to ensure that the services rendered to patients are, and are perceived to be, of acceptable quality.

Those who pay for health care services must hold managers of hospitals responsible for cost containment and for quality of care. Patients do sometimes pay directly for health care services, but even in the United States, direct payments by users accounted for just under 18% of total health spending in 1993.[1] By far the most important payers are collective funds, which can be either government or private insurance of some kind. They are both in the position to say what they expect of managers. In turn, managers have come to appreciate quality control programs as a way to indicate what they expect of physicians, nurses and other immediate providers of health care.

The concept of quality control of health care is conventionally traced back to 1863, when Florence Nightingale wrote about the causes of strikingly different death rates in hospitals in and outside London. Later, a surgeon at Massachusetts General Hospital in Boston, Ernest Amory Codman, pioneered quality control in the United States by suggesting in the early 1900s that surgeons should systematically gather the outcomes of their surgical procedures and care and make this information publicly known so that future patients might make informed decisions in selecting their own surgeons (Commission on Accreditation of Health Care Organizations, Agenda for Change, as cited in reference [2]).

In most of the 20th century, if attempts at quality control were made at all, they were based on auditing individual case histories, usually to explain why something had gone wrong. The problem with this approach was that it too infrequently provided information that could lead to systematic improvements in provision of care. The good thing about it was that it was well suited to picking up most of the pertinent detail of what actually happens to patients. As an example, this is what Codman wrote as a medical audit of his own clinical work (as cited in reference [2]):

> December 9, 1912. Female 59. Recurrent attack of gallstone colic. Cholecystectomy, appendectomy. Complications — none. 1916 letter: continued attacks of pain. April 17, 1917. Reentry for persistent biliary colic. Operators (E. A. C. and G. F. L., jr.). Gallstone removed, cystic duct tied off. Postoperative pain, jaundice, death on the seventh day. I was so sure I had done the operation correctly that I never once suspected the true cause of the unusual condition — division and ligation of the hepatic duct. A post-mortem examination through the incision showed the hepatic duct lay free in the wound. There was a tie on the proximal end of hepatic duct where I remembered having placed one at the time of the hemorrhage and had supposed the duct was a vein. In other words, I made

an error of skill (E-s) of the most gross character and even failed to recognize that I had made it (E-j). More than that, I would not have believed it, unless I had made the post-mortem myself and seen it with my own eyes. Hyperdistension of the duct had pushed off the tie, I think the patient died of pneumonia, but she could not have lived with a divided hepatic duct.

Codman had made a mistake during the second operation in 1917. The mistake is easy to understand for anyone who has ever seen how difficult it is to operate on the part of the liver facing obliquely down into the abdomen and back toward the spine. Bleeding occurred, and again, if you had seen an operation of this sort, you would wonder how surgeons ever manage to avoid bleeding. This one probably completely obscured Codman's already limited view of the operating field, and he had to stop it by tying one of the many small veins surrounding the hepatic duct. By mistake he also tied the hepatic duct, through which bile begins its flow from the liver to the small intestine. Bile cannot leave the liver if the hepatic duct is closed. When the liver becomes distended with bile, some of it leaks into the blood stream, and the patient dies.

It is a fallacy to think that mistakes can be completely avoided. No two patients are alike. Unless physicians avoid patients, they cannot avoid mistakes when treating patients. Responsible physicians make mistakes, because they treat patients. That's how it should be, but physicians must be able and willing to acknowledge mistakes, to learn from them, and to avoid as many of them as possible in the future. The efforts to make clinical decisions well should be predicated on a culture of self-scrutiny, sometimes by the physician himself as exemplified by Codman, but usually by other physicians facing the same challenges in their daily work.

To the extent that quality control was exercised at all, it was based on self-scrutiny, also termed medical audit, until the late 20th century. This began to change as leaders in health care became convinced that methods developed in clinical science and epidemiology could be adapted to a form of quality control that could be applied more systematically. That kind of quality control had been developed in industry, where W. Edwards Deming, an American statistician and educator, in the 1930s helped to develop and disseminate the statistical and managerial techniques necessary to monitor and improve quality of industrial production.[2] The adoption of Deming's ideas in the 1950s helped Japanese industry to near-dominance of world markets for a wide range of commodities. Adaptation of these principles to health care systems seemed to be possible because of two major advances.

One was the advent of the methodology of clinical science and epidemiology, especially statistical methods and computerized clinical databases. The latter opened the way for the routine storage of huge amounts of data concerning diseases and medical procedures. Although not yet fully satisfactory, the computerized patient record allows data from daily clinical work to be entered directly into the hospital database. The database can then be used for several purposes. First, as more data are entered by different physicians, the computer will accumulate information about any one patient in the system, and proponents hope that it will bring those data together to create a form of computer consciousness about the patient that physicians can use in their treatment of him or her. Secondly, the computer will accumulate information that some physicians and managers believe will help them to a better scientific understanding of the course of different diseases. Finally, the computer will enable hospital managers to monitor continuously what they believe are the quantity and quality of services, just as major department stores now monitor every item from the time it is received from the supplier until it is sold to a customer. For reasons to be given a little later, I believe that all three ideas are fundamentally flawed.

The other advance was the development of recommendations, guidelines and, ultimately, standards of care. To a large extent, guidelines are derived from the results of clinical science, especially the randomized clinical trial. They are often embodied in guideline-documents, which typically are quite lengthy reports prepared by experts on behalf of a medical society or a government agency. The reports must reflect not only what is known from clinical science about the prevention, diagnosis or treatment of the disease in question. They must also take into account what is feasible in practical clinical terms as well as in organizational and economic terms. The way such guideline-documents are prepared has itself turned into an academic discipline.[3]

A few years ago, I represented the European Atherosclerosis Society in a collaboration with other European scientific societies in drawing up recommendations for European physicians about preventing coronary artery disease. A major concern was the necessity for recommendations that would be meaningful for specialists as well as for general practitioners, for the poorly funded systems of health care in some former socialist countries of Eastern Europe as well as for the well funded systems of Western Europe, and for those parts of Europe where the disease is very common as well as for those parts where it is less common. We met regularly in London to spend a day discussing drafts, drinking tea and eating snacks less than ideal for preventing coronary artery disease.

There were six of us, each with some form of expertise in one or more aspects of the disease. We were all physicians, and we all worked with patients on a daily basis. One of the things we wrote a few times in the document was this: *"Ultimately, however, the decision to be made depends on clinical judgment"*. Another thing we wrote a few times was this: *"Physicians treat patients, not risk factors"*. Perhaps we should have written both much more frequently, because guidelines-documents are read not only by physicians who know how to take care of patients. They are also read by administrators, by representatives of industry, sometimes by politicians and perhaps increasingly by lawyers. The concern is that recommendations for how to take care of patients are interpreted by non-physicians as standards of care from which there should be as little departure as possible.

Managing Doctors

Many older physicians are deeply unhappy about the industrialization of medicine and the demise of clinical skills and the medical professional,[4] but for the most part, their articles and books cut no ice with managers and physician managers. That is because anything less than formal arguments on behalf of clinical skills and expertise are dismissed as sentimentality. Formal arguments, on the other hand, cannot be dismissed without formal counter-arguments. As it happens, formal arguments in defense of diversity and intuition have emerged, not from medicine, but from the realm of social and political studies.

What, if anything, is wrong with systems that ensure the quality of health care? What, if anything, is wrong with monitoring the behavior of health care workers? The answer, in brief, is that the quality control systems used in our health care systems, in principle as well as in practice, are able to gauge only the lower levels of human behavior. They are in principle and practice unable to measure human behavior on higher levels, but our health care systems depend on the adequacy of human behavior on higher as well as lower levels.

What is meant by lower and higher levels? I hasten to emphasize that I am not writing about levels of behavior requiring lesser or greater degrees of intelligence. Rather, behavior at lower levels can be described in the rational terms of degree of adherence to standards, instructions, algorithms, or any other kinds of description of procedures. Behavior at higher levels transcends such standards and descriptions, because it is a function of expertise.

As an example, the procedure for preparing an anesthesiology table for an operation can be described in rational terms: the oxygen hose must be connected to the oxygen outlet, and the hose for the anesthetic gas must be connected to the outlet for the anesthetic gas. The two should not be switched around. That procedure is in principle analogous to the procedure that a pilot must follow in preparing his aircraft for take-off. It can be adequately described in a handbook of standards, and the human behavior necessary to perform the procedure is transparently rational. That is what I mean by low level human behavior. It lends itself to monitoring in current quality control programs.

In contrast, what the anesthesiologist does during the operation itself cannot be adequately prescribed in a manual. For sure, the beginning anesthesiologist will roughly follow a procedure as described in textbooks of anesthesiology, but the beginner does not cope well with the many complex situations that arise during the course of surgery. Coping well requires experience, and the experienced anesthesiologist will do things during the operation that could not have been anticipated in any set of written instructions. He does so because experience has taught him how to anticipate fluctuations in blood pressure, how to anticipate how well the patient's blood is being oxygenated and how to anticipate a myriad of other details of the patient's progress through the operation. The patient who is critically ill would be ill served if all the anesthesiologist knew was a prescription, however detailed. Fortunately the anesthesiologist knows much more than that. He anticipates problems and he acts on the basis of intuition and experience. An experienced pilot does the same thing, and we like to be flown by experienced pilots. Only pilots with a crude sense of humor announce that take-off will be delayed until the instruction manual is on board.

This argument might seem obvious, but the importance of expertise and intuition has somehow managed to get itself lost on planners of our health care systems. I therefore venture to make the argument anyway, if only to emphasize that even an obvious argument can be stated in formal terms that must be formally refuted if it is to be dismissed. Hubert Dreyfus and Stuart Dreyfus (as cited in reference [5]) list several levels of competence from the beginner to the expert. The beginner must learn rules to follow in his first attempts, for example to drive a car. Everything he does at this stage is conscious, and his actions are explicitly consistent with instructions for applying brakes, changing gears and driving through traffic. As he progresses from beginner through increasing levels of competence and perhaps to expert racing driver, his actions depend less on remembering rules of driving and more on intuition and experience. Fast reactions are intuitive and reflexive, and they transcend explicit instructions.

A problem for planners of the health care systems, or of any human organizations, is that they cannot explicitly account for the expertise on which they depend. In health care, that expertise cannot be captured in the models of computerized quality assurance programs except as a "black box" of factors producing unpredictable variation, for example in the kind and amount of services rendered to patients. Yet to insist on meticulous adherence to standards, instructions and attention to rules would result in performance on the level of the beginner. For sure, it would be predictable and invariant, but it would be less than competent and much less than expert. It is not what patients expect. There is a qualitative leap from the level of the beginner to the level of the expert in all forms of human learning.

Bent Flyvbjerg makes these points in an analysis of political decisions and sociological theory.[5] His discussion is closely related to one of the themes of this book: the qualitative differences in the methods that we must use to understand different levels of complexity. In the case of sociology, Flyvbjerg argues that it is now high time for sociologists to bring to a conclusion the two hundred years of vain efforts exerted in order to formulate general theories of human behavior with the same predictive power as those of the natural sciences. Whereas Newton's theory of gravitation permits engineers to calculate how to put telecommunications satellites in orbit around the Earth, the bankruptcy of communism is only the most recent and sorrowful example of the failure of sociological theory to predict human behavior and the greater course of human events. According to Flyvbjerg, sociologists — and management of the health care systems is an application of a particular sociological theory — must give up the quest for rational laws of human behavior in favor of pragmatic approaches, varying from one context to another, that accept and take into account complexities of human behavior transcending the transparently rational. For example, the approaches necessary to understand what happened in urban planning in a particular city in Denmark will be inappropriate to an understanding of legislation concerning hand guns in California. All general theories of human social behavior, of which Marxist theory is just one example, should be greeted with skepticism.

Another theory of this sort is that the expert human behavior necessary to diagnose and treat patients with a great diversity of clinical problems can be directed according to principles developed for the automobile industry, understood and evaluated by the methods of clinical epidemiology, and modified as needed to meet the requirements of computers. New as well as very old observations suggest that this idea is likely to be very wrong indeed. What happens instead is that expertise and creativity are diverted from diagnosis and treatment of patients to the manipulation of and survival in great bureaucratic systems.

As examples, let us consider three related phenomena: transfer of high-risk patients, manipulation of perceptions of quality of care, and circumvention of rules of management to provide good care of patients.

Transferring High Risk Patients

In the 1860s, this is what Florence Nightingale wrote about transfers of high-risk patients:

> We have known incurable cases discharged from one hospital, to which deaths ought to have been accounted and received into another hospital, to die there in a day or two after admission, thereby lowering the mortality rate of the first at the expense of the second (as cited in reference [6]).

Transfer of high-risk patients from one hospital to another with the purpose of shifting responsibility for a poor outcome can also happen today, almost 140 years after Nightingale's study. The purpose can be to accommodate patient perceptions of quality of treatment. For example, physicians caring for or operating upon patients at private as well as public hospitals must consider seeing low-risk patients in the former and high risk patients in the latter setting, because the private hospital is financially more vulnerable to changing perceptions of performance. This can also happen as a result of the establishment of quality control programs, because the transfer of patients to other hospitals or to other patient categories can help to ensure that the program is associated with apparent improvements in patient outcomes.[7] It is more proper to make adjustments for degrees of illness, but departments and hospitals do not always trust the completeness of such adjustments, and some of them can be tempted to direct patient flows as they deem most expedient.

Physicians must, as individuals, also take rational precautions. Databases make it possible to monitor not only the performance of hospitals and departments, but also the performance of individual physicians. Physician-specific data are entered into score-cards so that patients can see which physicians, e.g. surgeons, have the highest and lowest rates of complications and successes. Any physician concerned about his and his family's future must take that into account when deciding whether to take on a high-risk patient, leave the job to someone else or identify a contra-indication to the procedure. Physicians take precautions. They are only human. The overall result is that physicians will sometimes choose to avoid those patients who need them most.

The Importance of Perceptions

Not all is what it appears to be. To ensure that hospitals are seen to be providing value for money, administrators must analyze the components of value and consider which components they can most efficiently improve. There are three components of value: clinical outcomes, costs and patient satisfaction, and they are not necessarily related. In one study, there was an unexpected inverse relationship between hospital costs and outcomes of coronary artery surgery. Contrary to expectations, the departments with the lowest costs tended to achieve the best outcomes.[6]

Outcomes are also not necessarily related to patient satisfaction. As a medical student I worked in several different departments of surgery. The surgeon who was most popular with his patients did not operate very well. His operations were in fact often alarmingly unsuccessful, but patients loved him, because he seemed to give them his undivided attention, recalled the names of their grandchildren, held their hands and stroked their hair. The surgeon who mastered diagnosis and did by far the most competent work in the operating theater was aloof if not arrogant, and patients feared and disliked him. Again, had they been measured, patient satisfaction and clinical outcomes including deaths would have been inversely related to each other. What you see is not always what you get. Doctors have always known that.

These relationships are not lost on managers of hospitals and health care plans, whether or not they depend on patient subscriptions. In whatever political system, focus on quality of care means that no hospital or health care plan can afford to ignore outcomes, costs or patient satisfaction. They have learned what management of airlines has known for decades. The most nebulous of the three, patient satisfaction can be easily manipulated, and it can be quantified in monetary terms. In an article with the perfectly serious title, *"The Economic Value of Caring"*, Issel and Kahn show how the "caring behavior" of health care professionals can affect the finances of a health care organization.[8] Appearances and perceptions, however illusory, have become an important currency of health care management.

Getting Around the Rules

Despite the importance attached to appearances, most physicians want to deliver sound medical care. That can often not be done, however, unless they circumvent guidelines for the management of patients that have become virtually and even explicitly mandatory. A survey of 1,124 practicing physicians in the United States showed that 39% exaggerated the severity of patient illness, changed billing diagnoses or reported symptoms that patients did not have so that patients could receive the care that the physicians believed was necessary.[9]

I asked a young hospital physician in San Francisco what she did when the insurance company would not approve a procedure she thought the patient needed. "I lie, of course," she said. "All good doctors lie".

What is the common denominator of avoidance of the sickest patients by hospitals and individual physicians, emphasis on perceptions rather than the reality of work by competent physicians, and the necessity of circumventing the rules of management to provide competent care? It is the deflection of intelligence, diligence and competence from work with patients to the interminable machinations necessary for survival in great bureaucracies. For physicians, it is an ignominious retreat from the work, skills and expertise of clinical medicine into petty preoccupation with the manipulation of a modern health care system.

Clinical Data Bases

Important and alarming as such physician behavior might be, it is less serious than a less obvious problem. The problem is the idea that the way physicians think of patients can somehow be transferred into a computerized data base. The idea comes from the randomized clinical trial, but we are all familiar with similar transfers of data concerning our money into databases belonging to the tax authorities or the bank. They enable the accountant to serve you quickly when you visit the bank, and they allow the tax authorities to know the insides of your pockets. No one would suggest that the bank accountant or the tax authorities should instead have committed to memory or ledger all of your mutual transactions. Computers store data of this sort quite well. They store similarly well patient data such as date of birth, family history, allergies, hospitalization dates, procedures performed and laboratory measurements. They can quite easily store thousands of bits of information about any particular patient. After all, that is what is done in all state-of-the-art clinical trials. So what is the problem? Well, there are really two problems.

One problem is that even very simple data — dates of birth and hospitalizations for example — must be as rigorously controlled for accuracy before they are entered into routine clinical databases, as they are when they are entered into the databases of randomized clinical trials, the model for the clinical data base. It is not a trivial task, however, and it is extremely time-consuming and expensive. If rigorous control is not exerted however, the clinical database will be worse than useless, because it will lead everyone astray. It will be garbage that comes out if it was garbage that went in. Garbage in, garbage out. That is the reason that entering data and keeping track of only a hundred patients in a clinical trial requires a full time project nurse. In a department of medicine that admits several thousand patients per year, proper entry of even a very limited number of data would require at least 10 full-time nurses. Very few hospital administrators can spend so much money on quality control programs, and most of the programs will therefore produce garbage.

The other problem is that a patient cannot in any meaningful way be reduced to a set of only 500 variables. Five hundred variables do not adequately characterize any patient, but even this number exceeds what is possible to collect for most quality assurance programs. This brings us back to a dichotomy that I shall attempt to discuss in the rest of this chapter.

Categories of Patients and Disease

For people who do not, and who are not supposed to take care of patients, it can be difficult to keep in mind a fundamental dichotomy and balance that everyone recognizes in principle. In clinical medicine, it is the dichotomy between patients and categories of patients, between clinical diversity and the principles and generalities of clinical medicine. But really, it is the dichotomy that I have discussed several times earlier in this book. In genetics, it is the tension between the biometric and the Mendelian approaches to understanding evolution, and in philosophy, it is the difference between

Aristotelian empiricism and Platonic idealism. In scientific philosophy, it is the balance between complexity theory and reductionism, and in everyday life, it's the balance between the joy of the infinite details of geology and life on a mountain side and the equal joy of contemplating the mountain in the distance as the "mother of all mountains".

Our present approach to quality of health care is no longer balanced. The balance has been shifted in favor of categories and generalities. They receive our attention, and we have forgotten about clinical diversity. There are numerous problems with this unbalanced approach. I'll discuss three.

Communication

First, in order to communicate, physicians, administrators and database managers must speak the same language. Details of patient management must somehow be reduced and classified for entry into the database. The International Classification of Disease (ICD) codes are commonly used for this purpose. When compared to patient records, however, there was a serious loss of pertinent information when it was classified as ICD-9 codes.[7] The codes captured only 67% of the diagnostic information, only 36% of the clinical findings, and only 40% of the treatments and procedures. The failure of coding systems to capture concepts documented to be part of real clinical care is a very serious problem if clinical databases are to be used not only for research but also for assessment of quality of care.

Clinical Diversity and Clinical Decisions

Secondly, the most serious aspect of the contemporary approach to quality of care is that it does not balance well between the nature of clinical care, which is complex, and the requirements of management, which in comparison are simple. The approach reduces clinical complexity and diversity to a few large categories of diseases that can be managed by current methods of computerized quality assessment. Coronary artery disease is as good an example as any. It is not one disease, and it can be confused with several other diseases. Let me give a few examples.

Most patients do not go to their doctor or to the hospital with the correct diagnosis written on a sign pinned to their chest. They come because they have chest pain, and the physician must find out whether it is due to closure of a coronary artery and resulting myocardial infarction, or whether it might be due to something quite different. Some of the other causes of chest pain are much less dangerous than myocardial infarction, and at least one of them is more dangerous.

Pericarditis is an example of a disease that is usually less dangerous than myocardial infarction. It is an inflammation of a thin moistured sac called the pericardium that envelops the heart in the chest cavity. Pericarditis is quite common, and it can usually be treated quite adequately with a mild pain killer like aspirin. A patient with pericarditis can be thought to have myocardial infarction, however. The changes in the electrocardiogram caused by pericarditis and myocardial infarction can, at a particular stage in each disease, resemble each other closely.

Instead of emphasizing the ability of physicians to differentiate between patients with different causes of chest pain, however, we currently emphasize speed in treating patients with one of those causes of chest pain, myocardial infarction. For many patients treatment includes aspirin and either a thrombolytic drug or removal of the clot with a catheter. Aspirin and thrombolytic drugs can dissolve clots in the coronary arteries, but they can also necessarily dissolve any clots that might have formed to stop bleeding from other blood vessels in the body. They can therefore cause bleeding from those other blood vessels. The risk of bleeding is worth running if you have a myocardial infarction, because, taken together, the two drugs can reduce the death rate from 13% to 8%.[10] It is not worth running, on the other hand, if you only have pericarditis, because patients with pericarditis do not usually die. If a patient with pericarditis is given a thrombolytic drug by mistake, however, the inflamed pericardium can bleed so severely that it prevents the pumping action of the heart. Then the patient might die. The drug can also cause a bleeding into the brain, a cerebral hemorrhage, which can be permanently disabling. It can also kill the patient.

Other causes of chest pain are more dangerous than myocardial infarction. An example is dissection of the aorta. The aorta is the largest artery in the body. The heart pumps blood directly into the aorta after the blood has been oxygenated in the lungs. Sometimes a small hole in the innermost layer of the wall of the aorta allows blood under high pressure to enter into the aortic wall itself, splitting apart and dissecting its way between the layers of the wall. The dissection can extend into the arteries that branch off from the aorta. Sometimes the bleeding into the wall stops because the blood in the wall coagulates, forming a protective clot, but at other times the patient dies, either because the artery has been closed off by the accumulation of blood in the wall, or because the artery has burst so that the heart pumps blood almost directly into the cavity of the chest or the abdomen. Dissection of the aorta causes changes in the electrocardiogram that can also mimic a myocardial infarction, and the physician can be led to think that the chest pain is due to a myocardial infarction. If he gives the patient a thrombolytic drug, it will increase the bleeding, and it will probably kill the patient.

There are about 10 conditions that a physician routinely must consider as causes of chest pain before he decides that the patient has myocardial infarction and treats him or her with drugs to dissolve clots. You might therefore expect that assessments of the quality of care of patients with chest pain were focused on that particularly crucial stage in the diagnosis and treatment of the disease, whatever it might be. That's not the case. The most commonly employed measurements of the quality of care of patients with myocardial infarction have been the death rate and the "door-to-needle time" or the "door-to-balloon time." The door-to-needle time is the time elapsed from the arrival of the patient at the hospital until the thrombolytic drug is infused into a vein in the arm, and the door-to-balloon-time is the time from arrival to inflation of the balloon in the segment of the coronary artery that has been closed by a clot.

Deaths and door-to-needle or door-to-balloon times are used because they are simple to measure. One of many problems is that they ignore whether differential diagnosis has been adequately handled. If patients with pericarditis or dissection of the aorta have been mistakenly treated with a drug to dissolve clots, those mistakes would not be entered into the quality assessment data base, because the patients did not have myocardial infarction. They would, in other words, not pertain to the series of patients with myocardial infarction, and the "indicators" of the quality of care of patients with myocardial infarction, i.e. death rates and door-to-needle or door-to-balloon times, would not reflect lapses of quality that are much more important than getting the patient from "door to needle" within 15 or 30 minutes.

The way to solve this problem is to focus attention on patient diversity, in this case on all of the patients with chest pain, rather than on only one diagnostic category of patients, in this case those patients who really did have myocardial infarction. We should have an even broader view, however. If we are to assess the quality of diagnosis and treatment, that assessment must be accorded all or a random sample of all patients treated by a hospital, a department or a physician, and not only the patients belonging to one or a few categories. Although categorization is convenient and probably necessary for databases that currently available computers can handle, it inevitably misleads physicians, managers and payers. A better alternative is to do systematic medical audits of a random sample of patients consecutively admitted to a hospital or a hospital department for whatever reason. We would all be better off if we did that. The size of the random sample of such patients can easily be adjusted to be in accordance with the amount of money available for the exercise. The reason that managers don't like that idea is that it does not lend itself to computerization and monitoring by non-physicians.

Clinical Diversity and Statistics

Thirdly, a deeper disquiet about this matter is due to the way we think about disease and categories of disease. In earlier chapters of this book we saw that lowering cholesterol in patients with coronary artery disease substantially increases their chances of survival. The proportion of patients with coronary artery disease and hypercholesterolemia placed on therapy with cholesterol-lowering diet or drugs could therefore be considered a measurement of the quality of care of these patients.[6] I have been a proponent of that strategy for many years, and on average it really is a good one. However, as we also have seen in earlier chapters, patients with coronary artery disease differ substantially, not only in their risk of dying within a few years of a myocardial infarction, but also in the degree to which they benefit from cholesterol-lowering treatment.

Patients with coronary artery disease therefore do not come from the same mold. They are all different, even if their coronary disease is due to atherosclerosis. To complicate matters even more, not all forms of coronary artery disease are due to atherosclerosis. Admittedly, atherosclerosis is the most common cause of narrowing of the arteries supplying the heart muscle, but those arteries can be narrowed by other diseases. The following are non-atherosclerotic causes of coronary artery disease: congenital abnormalities (e.g. stenoses, atresias, anomalous origins of a coronary artery), embolism (from natural or prosthetic aortic or mitral valves affected by thrombosis or infected by bacteria), and various forms of non-bacterial and non-atherosclerotic inflammation of the artery wall (e.g. Kawasaki disease, polyarteritis nodosa, lupus erythematosus disseminatus, Takayasu's disease) as well as syphilis. Some of these diseases are easy to distinguish from atherosclerotic coronary artery disease, but others are not, and treatment must be different. It is almost certain, however, that the standardization of medical practice increasingly required by those who formulate treatment policy means that some patients with non-atherosclerotic coronary artery disease are taking cholesterol-lowering drugs to no avail and, even worse, that they are not receiving the therapy relevant to the disease afflicting them.

The deeper disquiet that I referred to above is that our thinking about the range of diseases that may afflict us is too much anchored in concepts of classical epidemiology and statistics. The central concept here is the Gaussian distribution of values around an all-important mean value. That mean value can be approached by calculating the averages of several series of measurements. The more measurements, the closer the average values of them will approach the "true mean value" of the "true distribution of values". I use quotation marks to indicate that these are abstractions, like the "mother of all mountains." The average height of soldiers in World War I was lower than in World War II. The more measurements that were made before sending the young men to the battlefields, the more we know about the all important question of their mean height. That was okay, because height is normally distributed, and the distribution can be adequately characterized in terms of the mean and the variance.

Many biological distributions are not Gaussian, however. Instead, they are characterized by a few large values, a somewhat larger number of medium-sized values, and a large number of small values. To take an example, the heart pumps blood into the aorta, which is the body's largest artery. Like the trunk of a tree, it branches into an ever increasing number of smaller arteries until blood finally reaches the capillaries through millions of tiny arteries called arterioles. When things are distributed in this way, a mean value of the diameter of an artery does not make any sense, because it depends on how far out into the arterial tree you have decided to make your measurements. If you include measurements of millions of arterioles, the mean diameter will be very small indeed. On the other hand, if you include only the first three or four branchings, the mean diameter will be quite large.

A distribution of values of this kind is fractal rather than Gaussian. A fractal distribution cannot be characterized by a mean value. Instead, it is characterized by the number of small values relative to the number of large values. That characteristic is called the fractal dimension. Fractal distributions have been known for more than three hundred years by mathematicians interested in this particular kind of statistics, but they have not been employed in many studies of biological problems. That should change. For example, some disturbances of heart rhythm can best be understood in terms of a fractal distribution of intervals between attacks. Larry S. Liebovitch of Florida Atlantic University has explained fractal statistics well for biologists and simple physicians.[10]

Disease distributions are also fractal rather than Gaussian. They are fractal in two ways. First, a small number of diseases each affect a large number of patients (e.g. asthma, coronary artery disease, psoriasis, type II diabetes), a somewhat larger number of diseases each affect a somewhat smaller number of patients (e.g. claudication, type I diabetes, familial hypercholesterolemia) and a very large number of diseases each affect a very small number of patients (e.g. acromegaly, Creutzfeldt-Jakob disease, diabetes insipidus). Secondly, some of the diseases affecting a large number of patients can be subdivided into smaller and smaller subgroups. In the case of coronary artery disease, we already did that exercise a little earlier in this chapter, and it can be repeated for all the other diseases afflicting a large number of patients. It can also be done for each of the medium sized diseases, and even extremely rare diseases can be further subdivided into very extremely rare diseases.

One of the classic examples of a fractal distribution is the measurements of the length of a coastline. On a not too detailed map of California, the coast runs about 700 kilometers north from Los Angeles to San Francisco. On a more detailed map, however, it is easy to see that it is really about 2000 kilometers long, and if you measured it meter by meter, or centimeter by centimeter, following each nook and cranny, it would be far longer. In other words, the length of the coastline depends on the unit of measurement. It's the same with disease. The number of diseases depends on how closely you look.

Thinking in terms of a Gaussian distribution of diseases, however, makes us look for an "average patient" who somehow has the essential attributes of all of the patients of the distribution of patients of which he is the average (or the mean, if we are to be really correct). But just as there is no average diameter of the arteries in the body, there is no average patient. The average patient is an abstraction, like the mother of all mountains. He is a Platonic idea.

Variance in this context is a nuisance, and the less variance the better. Achieving as much homogeneity of patients' groups as possible is considered essential in clinical research as well as in the planning of health care systems. It can be legitimate in the case of research, because the purpose of clinical research can be to answer extremely simple questions such as *"Can lowering of cholesterol prevent atherosclerosis in humans as it does in monkeys?"* It is not legitimate in planning health care for routine patients, however, because they do not have simple problems. Some have a common disease that seems to fit into the algorithm, but many patients either have a combination of common diseases, or they have one of a huge number of rare diseases, or they have a combination of rare diseases, common diseases and a host of non-disease problems. It is essential for making sensible and humane medical decisions to distinguish all these cases, yet none of these problems or combinations of problems are adequately considered within the standards and algorithms that some managers seem to think physicians must follow.

There can be little doubt that disease distributions are fractal rather than Gaussian. When we use statistical concepts predicated on the Gaussian distribution, we are cramming patients into boxes they do not fit, and continuing to do so will be a source of chronic conflict in our health care systems. The conflict will continue to be between physicians, who know diversity, and managers including physician managers, for whom variation is inconvenient if not fundamentally incompatible with the categorizations of patient data required by the computers and database programs currently available. We are all going to be unhappy in this new world of medicine.

In contrast, thinking in terms of a fractal distribution of diseases makes us once again focus on the diversity of clinical experience. This will ring true in the ears of clinicians, and it is intuitively comprehensible for everyone including patients. The problem is that fractal statistics are not developed as well as those based on the Gaussian distribution, and the methodology of current quality control and health care management is predicated on Gaussian statistics. That is not primarily the fault of managers. Instead, those of us who are physicians and researchers should consider whether we have led managers into fallacious concepts and thinking about what hospitals are for. Rather than continuing to accept faulty reasoning, based on abstract principles such as the average, we should try to work out ways of monitoring how well we treat very different patients with a huge diversity of diseases including that huge group of diseases called coronary artery disease.

Conclusions

Diseases of the arteries, including disease of the arteries of the heart, *"did not suddenly leap into existence at the beginning of the 20th century, fully armed for destruction, like the Athena from the brow of Zeus."* [1] Instead, they have been with us for at least 3,500 years, perhaps since we began to drink the milk and eat the meat of domesticated animals about 10,000 years ago. During most of those many years, atherosclerotic and thrombotic diseases were not important, because most people were neither affluent nor sedentary enough to get them. Quite the reverse. Genetically programmed to eat fat whenever available in an environment of food scarcity, people who domesticated large mammals had better chances of survival. Of the few who were both affluent and sedentary, many probably still died of infectious or other diseases before the slow narrowing or sudden clogging of their arteries could make them sick or strike them down.

All this changed when industrialization and fossil fuels enabled farmers to raise huge numbers of livestock for meat and milk and enabled everyone to use their muscles less. Now, for the first time, several conditions, including the cultivation of tobacco, were simultaneously present, and ultimately they made "heart attack" a household word. Probably beginning in the late 19th century, disease due to atherosclerosis and thrombosis increased and peaked shortly after the middle of the 20th century in Western Europe, North America and the other established market economies. Thereafter it declined, but by the opening of the 21st century, that decline may have stopped at a stable, somewhat lower level than in the mid-century heyday of the disease. The epidemic has moved on to the developing countries of the world, which now are adopting, or being asked to adopt, the agricultural practices developed in Europe and North America in the 19th and 20th centuries. Farmers all over the Earth will raise more grain, not to feed their fellow citizens, but to feed animals from which the affluent among their fellow citizens will have milk and meat containing only 10% of the energy of the grain. This grossly inefficient way of producing food will increasingly be based on fossil fuel, deforestation and intensive tillage of the ever-thinning layer of topsoil.

Whereas Europe in the 18th century averted ecological catastrophe by the enlightened application of the technology then available, ecological recovery seems less likely now. That is not because agronomists now know less than they did then. Quite the contrary, but decisions are now not made by aristocrats with a vested interest in conservation of their estates. Rather they are made by vacillating governments under pressure from an intrepid food and agricultural industry. Even before the emergence of molecular genetics, 20th century breeding practices had resulted in biological uniformity and loss of that resilience without which plants or animals could not have emerged on Earth, and, in seeking to increase the yields of crops and to protect crops from pests, the new agricultural biotechnology only seems to deepen that loss of diversity. We might well appreciate these complex relationships, but as shareholders or workers in that industry, or even as supermarket customers, we seem to have no short term economic interest in less remunerative agricultural practices, however sustainable in the long term.

Atherosclerotic disease is preventable, and no one will deter those who so wish from preventing the disease by living wisely. The problem is that the food avoided by the wise will get into the stomachs of the unwise, and the unwise will continue to succumb to atherosclerotic and thrombotic disease. Increasingly elegant pharmaceutical, surgical and possibly gene-therapeutic or stem-cell-therapeutic solutions to the problem of heart disease will emerge from sophisticated biotechnological research, and one scenario is reliance on biotechnology and a heavy-handed system of industrialized medicine to bail us out of the consequences of diseases promoted by industrialized agriculture and our inadequate adaptation to life as city dwellers. In this scenario, agriculture, urbanization, the pharmaceutical industry and health care organizations constitute an integrated economic system of production and treatment of coronary artery disease.

The other scenario would be to emulate the European Enlightenment of the 18th century. That is a challenge for national governments, and it should be a challenge for international government on the continental level of the European Union and on the intercontinental level of the United Nations. Politicians channel large amounts of taxpayer money into income supports and subsidies for farmers, especially big farmers or agricultural industry. Before they hand over the money, however, politicians should be asked to think about the implications for the health of taxpayers when they discuss with farmers what should be farmed. As it spreads across the planet, coronary artery disease will be the leading cause of loss of years of good life by 2020, but it is just one of the unwanted consequences of agriculture that is subsidized to raising livestock and tobacco. Government must take responsibility for policies that are obviously related to human health,[2] but government must also integrate health policy with policies for science, industry, urban planning and agriculture.[3]

In a wider perspective, human health and life have always depended absolutely on the way our genes interact with the environment. With the introduction of agriculture ten thousand years ago, however, we began a process of fundamentally reshaping the world around us, and now we virtually decide our environment consciously with good intent, consciously with bad intent, out of ignorance, or by calamity and accident. The gross inefficiency of producing food by raising livestock, fed the grain that we could eat, is one of the mechanisms by which we are so efficiently wasting and destroying those resources of the earth that sustain us and must sustain our children. It's time to see what's happening on the fields and pastures just outside the hospitals in our global village, to encourage basic research in biological, agricultural and clinical diversity and complexity, and to renounce the political defeatism with which we closed the 20th century. We must once again develop the political will to fashion our rural and urban environments to protect nature and to promote human health and sanity.

References

Introduction

1. Enos, W. F., Holmes, R. H., & Beyer, J. (1953). Coronary disease among United States soldiers killed in action in Korea. *JAMA*, *152*. 1090–1093.
2. EU works with ESC on "Heart Plan for Europe" and strategies to tackle Europe's cardiovascular disease epidemic. European Society of Cardiology Press & PR Office. 11–7–2002. Internet Communication.
3. Guldet fra Moskva (2001). *Finansieringen af de nordiske kommunistpartier 1917–1990*. Copenhagen: Forum.
4. The Joint European Society of Cardiology/American College of Cardiology Committee (2000). Myocardial infarction redefined — A consensus document of The Joint European Society of Cardiology/American College of Cardiology Committee for the Redefinition of Myocardial Infarction. *European Heart Journal*, *21*, 1502–1513.

Chapter 1

1. Harper, A. E. (1996). Dietary guidelines in perspective. *The Journal of Nutrition*, *126*, 1042S–1048S.
2. Leibowitz, J. O. (1970). *The history of coronary heart disease*. London: Wellcome Institute of the History of Medicine.
3. Labarthe, D. R. (1998). *Epidemiology and prevention of cardiovascular diseases: A global challenge*. Gaithersburg, Maryland: Aspen Publishers, Inc.
4. Osler, W. (1897). *Lectures on Angina Pectoris and Allied States*. Edinburgh and London: Young J. Pentland.
5. Porter, R. (1997). *The greatest benefit to mankind. A medical history of humanity from antiquity to the present* (paperback 1999 ed.). London: HarperCollins.
6. Bizzozero J. (1882). Über einen neuen Formbestandteil des Blutes und dessen Rolle bei der Thrombose und der Blutgerinnung. *Virchow's Arch. Path. Anat. Physiol. Klin. Med.*, *90*, 261–332.
7. Dahlerup (1844). Society minutes. *Ugeskrift for Læger*, *10*, 214–218.
8. Osler, W. (1892). *The principles and practice of medicine: The classics of medicine library ed*. New York: D. Appleton and Company.

9. Herrick, J. B. (1912). Clinical features of sudden obstruction of the coronary arteries. *JAMA*, *59*, 2015–2020.

Chapter 2

1. Stallones, R. A. (1980). The rise and fall of ischemic heart disease. *Scientific American*, *243*, 53–59.
2. Malmros, H. (1950). The relation of nutrition to health: A statistical study of the effect of war-time on arteriosclerosis, cardiosclerosis, tuberculosis and diabetes. *Acta Med. Scand.*, *246*, 137–153.
3. Malmros, H. (1980). Diet, lipids and atherosclerosis. *Acta Med. Scand.*, *207*, 145–149.
4. Schettler, G. (1979). Cardiovascular diseases during and after World War II: A comparison of the Federal Republic of Germany with other European countries. *Prev. Med.*, *8*, 581–590.
5. Sijbrands, E. J. G., Westendorp, R. G. J., Defesche, J. C., De Meijer, P. H. E. M., Smelt, A. H. M., & Kastelein, J. P. (2001). Mortality over 2 centuries in large pedigree with familial hypercholesterolaemia; family tree mortality study. *BMJ*, *322*, 1019–1023.
6. Faergeman, O. (2001). The atherosclerosis epidemic: methodology, nosology, and clinical practice. *Am. J. Cardiol.*, *88* (2-A), 4E–7E.
7. McKay, J. P., Hill, B. D., & Buckler, J. (1999). The Revolution in Energy and Industry. In: A. Shaw, D. Anderson, L. Rothrauff, & C. M. Horn (Eds), *A history of western society* (Vol. C). *From the revolutionary era to the present* (pp. 724–753). Boston, New York: Houghton Mifflin Company.
8. Yusuf, S., Reddy, S., Ôunpuu, S., & Anand, S. (2001). Global burden of cardiovascular diseases. Part I: General considerations, the epidemiologic transition, risk factors, and impact of urbanization. *Circulation*, *104*, 2746–2753.
9. Tunstall-Pedoe, H., Kuulasmaa, K., Mähönen, M., Tolonen, H., Ruokokoski, E., & Amouyel, P. (1999). Contribution of trends in survival and coronary-event rates to changes in coronary heart disease mortality: 10-year results from 37 WHO MONICA Project populations. *Lancet*, *353*, 1547–1557.
10. Lawlor, D. A., Smith, G. D., Leon, D. A., Sterne, J. A., & Ebrahim, S. (2002). Secular trends in mortality by stroke subtype in the 20th century: a retrospective analysis. *Lancet*, *360* (9348), 1818–1823.
11. Wong, C. K., & White, H. D. (2002). Has the mortality rate from acute myocardial infarction fallen substantially in recent years? *Eur. Heart J.*, *23* (9), 689–692.
12. Wong, N. D., Wilson, P. W., & Kannel, W. B. (1991). Serum cholesterol as a prognostic factor after myocardial infarction: the Framingham Study. *Ann. Intern. Med.*, *115* (9), 687–693.
13. Solberg, L. A., & Strong, J. P. (1983). Risk factors and atherosclerotic lesions: A review of autopsy studies. *Arteriosclerosis*, *3*, 187–198.
14. Strong, J. P., Solberg, L. A., & Restrepo, C. (1968). Atherosclerosis in persons with coronary heart disease. *Laboratory Investigation*, *18*, 527–537.

15. Law, M. R., & Wald, N. (1999). Why heart disease mortality is low in France: The time lag explanation. *BMJ*, *318*, 1471–1476.
16. Doll, R., & Peto, R. (1981). The causes of cancer. *J. Natl. Cancer Inst.*, *66*, 1292–1305.
17. Drummond, J. C., Wilbraham, A., & Hollingsworth, D. (1957). *The Englishman's food: A history of five centuries of English diet*. Pimlico.
18. Harnack, L. J., Jeffery, R. W., & Boutelle, K. N. (2000). Temporal trends in energy intake in the United States: an ecologic perspective. *Am. J. Clin. Nutr.*, *71* (6), 1478–1484.
19. O'Keefe, S. F. (2000). Animal, marine, and vegetable oils. In: K. F. Kiple, & K. C. Ornelas (Eds), *The Cambridge world history of food* (pp. 375–388). Cambridge: Cambridge University Press.
20. Johnson, C. L., Rifkind, B. M., Sempos, C. T., Carroll, M. D., Bachorik, P. S., & Briefel, R. R. *et al.* (1993). Declining serum total cholesterol levels among U.S. adults: The National Health and Nutrition Examination Surveys. *JAMA*, *269* (23), 3002–3008.
21. Langvad, J. (2002). Personal communication.
22. Morris, J. N. (1951). Recent history of coronary disease. *Lancet*, *1* (1), 69–70, 73.
23. Leibowitz, J. O. (1970). *The history of coronary heart disease*. London, Wellcome Institute of the History of Medicine.
24. Bucher, H. C., Griffith, L. E., & Guyatt, G. H. (1999). Systematic review on the risk and benefit of different cholesterol-lowering interventions. *Arterioscler. Thromb. Vasc. Biol.*, *19* (2), 187–195.
25. Heart Protection Study Collaborative Group (2002). MRC/BHF Heart Protection Study: Randomised placebo-controlled trial of cholesterol lowering with simvastatin in 20,536 high-risk individuals: A randomised placebo-controlled trial. *Lancet*, *360*, 7–22.
26. Libby, P., Hansson, G. K., & Pober, J. S. (1999). Atherogenesis and inflammation. In: K. R. Chien (Ed.), *Molecular basis of cardiovascular disease* (pp. 349–366). Philadelphia: W. B. Saunders Company.
27. Pearson, T. A. (1999). Threats to the continued decline in cardiovascular disease in the United States. *Circulation*, *100* (18), IA.
28. The Joint European Society of Cardiology/American College of Cardiology Committee (2000). Myocardial infarction redefined — A consensus document of The Joint European Society of Cardiology/American College of Cardiology Committee for the Redefinition of Myocardial Infarction. *European Heart Journal*, *21*, 1502–1513.
29. Jensen, J. M., Gerdes, L. U., Jensen, H. K., Christiansen, T. M., Brorholt-Petersen, J. U., & Faergeman, O. (2000). Association of coronary heart disease with age-adjusted aortocoronary calcification in patients with familial hypercholesterolaemia. *J. Intern. Med.*, *247* (4), 479–484.

Chapter 3

1. Impending Global Pandemic of Cardiovascular Diseases (1999). *Challenges and opportunities for the prevention and control of cardiovascular diseases in developing countries and economies in transition.* Barcelona, Philadelphia: Prous Science.
2. EU works with ESC on "Heart Plan for Europe" and strategies to tackle Europe's cardiovascular disease epidemic. European Society of Cardiology Press & PR Office. 11–7–2002. Internet Communication.
3. *The Global Burden of Disease* (1996). Cambridge: Harvard University Press.
4. Yusuf, S., Reddy, S., Ôunpuu, S., Anand, S. (2001). Global burden of cardiovascular diseases. Part I: General considerations, the epidemiologic transition, risk factors, and impact of urbanization. *Circulation, 104*, 2746–2753.
5. Yusuf, S., Reddy, S., Ôunpuu, S., & Anand, S. (2001). Global burden of cardiovascular diseases. Part II: Variations in cardiovascular disease by specific ethnic groups and geographic regions and prevention strategies. *Circulation, 104*, 2855–2864.
6. The World Health Report 2002 (2002). *Reducing risks, promoting health life.* Geneva: World Health Organization.
7. Brown, M. S., & Goldstein, J. L. (1996). Heart attacks: gone with the century? *Science, 272*, 629.
8. World Agriculture: Towards 2010 (1995). *An FAO Study.* Chichester, New York, Brisbane, Toronto, Singapore: Food and Agricultural Organization of the United Nations and John Wiley & Sons, 1995.

Chapter 4

1. Anitschkow, N. N. (1933). A history of experimentation on arterial atherosclerosis in animals. In: H. T. Blumenthal (Ed.), *Cowdry's Arteriosclerosis. A Survey of the Problem* (pp. 21–44). Springfield, Illinois, USA: Charles C. Thomas.
2. Thannhauser, S. J., & Magendantz, H. (1937). The different clinical groups of xanthomatous diseases; a clinical physiological study of 22 cases. *Annals of Internal Medicine, 11*, 1662–1746.
3. Müller, C. (1939). Angina pectoris in hereditary xanthomatosis. *Arch. Int. Med., 64*, 675–700.
4. Brown, M. S., & Goldstein, J. L. (1986). A receptor-mediated pathway for cholesterol homeostasis. *Science, 232* (4746), 34–47.
5. Poulter, N. R., & Chapman, N. (1999). Epidemiology of Atherosclerosis. In: D. J. Betteridge, D. R. Illingworth, & J. Shepherd (Eds). *Lipoproteins in health and disease* (pp. 541–573). London, Sydney, Auckland: Arnold.
6. Enos, W. F., Holmes, R. H., & Beyer, J. (1953). Coronary disease among United States soldiers killed in action in Korea. *JAMA, 152*, 1090–1093.

7. Law, M. R., Wald, N. J., & McGill, H. C. Jr. (1994). By how much and how quickly does reduction in serum cholesterol concentrations lower risk of ischaemic heart disease. *BMJ*, *308*, 367–372.

8. Corr, L. A., & Oliver, M. F. (1997). The low fat/low cholesterol diet is ineffective. *Eur. Heart J.*, *18* (1), 18–22.

9. Bucher, H. C., Griffith, L. E., & Guyatt, G. H. (1999). Systematic review on the risk and benefit of different cholesterol-lowering interventions. *Arterioscler. Thromb. Vasc. Biol.*, *19* (2), 187–195.

10. Turpeinen, O., Karvonen, M. J., Pekkarinen, M., Miettinen, M., Elosuo, R., & Paavilainen, E. (1979). Dietary prevention of coronary heart disease: The Finnish Mental Hospital Study. *Int. J. Epidemiol.*, *8* (2), 99–118.

11. Hjermann, I., Velve, B. K., Holme, I., & Leren, P. (1981). Effect of diet and smoking intervention on the incidence of coronary heart disease: Report from the Oslo Study Group of a randomised trial in healthy men. *Lancet*, *2* (8259), 1303–1310.

12. Burr, M. L., Fehily, A. M., Gilbert, J. F., Rogers, S., Holliday, R. M., & Sweetnam, P. M. *et al.* (1989). Effects of changes in fat, fish, and fibre intakes on death and myocardial reinfarction: Diet and Reinfarction Trial (DART). *Lancet*, *2* (8666), 757–761.

13. de Lorgeril, M., Renaud, S., Mamelle, N., Salen, P., Martin, J. L., & Monjaud, I. *et al.* (1994). Mediterranean alpha-linolenic acid-rich diet in secondary prevention of coronary heart disease. *Lancet*, *343*, 1454–1459.

14. Oliver, M. F. (2000). Pioneer research in Britain into atherosclerosis and coronary heart disease — an historical review. *Atherosclerosis*, *150*, 1–12.

15. The Lipid Research Clinics Coronary Primary Prevention Trial Results (1984). I. Reduction in incidence of coronary heart disease. *JAMA*, *251* (3), 351–364.

16. The Lipid Research Clinics Coronary Primary Prevention Trial Results (1984). II. The relationship of reduction in incidence of coronary heart disease to cholesterol lowering. *JAMA*, *251* (3), 365–374.

17. Scandinavian Simvastatin Survival Study Group (1994). Randomised trial of cholesterol lowering in 4444 patients with coronary heart disease: The Scandinavian Simvastatin Survival Study (4S). *Lancet*, *344* (8934), 1383–1389.

18. Sacks, F. M., Pfeffer, M. A., Moye, L. A., Rouleau, J. L., Rutherford, J. D., & Cole, T. G. *et al.* (1996). The effect of pravastatin on coronary events after myocardial infarction in patients with average cholesterol levels: Cholesterol and Recurrent Events Trial investigators. *N. Engl. J. Med.*, *335* (14), 1001–1009.

19. The Long-Term Intervention with Pravastatin in Ischaemic Disease (LIPID) Study Group (1998). Prevention of cardiovascular events and death with pravastatin in patients with coronary heart disease and a broad range of initial cholesterol levels. *N. Engl. J. Med.*, *339* (19), 1349–1357.

20. Shepherd, J., Cobbe, S. M., Ford, I., Isles, C. G., Lorimer, A. R., & MacFarlane, P. W. *et al.* (1995). Prevention of coronary heart disease with pravastatin in men with hypercholesterolemia. West of Scotland Coronary Prevention Study Group. *N. Engl. J. Med.*, *333* (20), 1301–1307.

21. Downs, J. R., Clearfield, M., Weis, S., Whitney, E., Shapiro, D. R., Beere, P. A. *et al.* (1998). Primary prevention of acute coronary events with lovastatin in men and women with average cholesterol levels: results of AFCAPS/TexCAPS: Air Force/ Texas Coronary Atherosclerosis Prevention Study. *JAMA, 279* (20), 1615–1622.
22. Heart Protection Study Collaborative Group (2002). MRC/BHF Heart Protection Study: Randomised placebo-controlled trial of cholesterol lowering with simvastatin in 20,536 high-risk individuals: A randomised placebo-controlled trial. *Lancet, 360*, 7–22.
23. Rubins, H. B., Robins, S. J., Collins, D., Fye, C. L., Anderson, J. W., Elam, M. B. *et al.* (1999). Gemfibrozil for the secondary prevention of coronary heart disease in men with low levels of high-density lipoprotein cholesterol. *New England Journal of Medicine, 341*, 410–418.
24. The BIP Study Group (2000). Secondary prevention by raising HDL cholesterol and reducing triglycerides in patients with coronary artery disease: The Bezafibrate Infarction Prevention (BIP) Study. *Circulation, 102*, 21–27.
25. Nestle, M. (2002). *Food politics: How the food industry influences nutrition and health*. Berkeley: University of California Press.

Chapter 5

1. Menotti, A., Kromhout, D., Blackburn, H., Fidanza, F., Buzina, R., & Nissinen, A. (1999). Food intake patterns and the 25-year mortality from coronary heart disease: Cross-cultural correlations in the Seven Countries Study: The Seven Countries Study Reseach Group. *European Journal of Epidemiology, 15*, 507–515.
2. Burr, M. L., Fehily, A. M., Gilbert, J. F., Rogers, S., Holliday, R. M., & Sweetnam, P. M. *et al.* (1989). Effects of changes in fat, fish, and fibre intakes on death and myocardial reinfarction: Diet and Reinfarction Trial (DART). *Lancet, 2* (8666), 757–761.
3. Singh, R. B., Rastogi, S. S., Verma, R., Laxmi, B., Singh, R., & Ghosh, S. *et al.* (1992). Randomised controlled trial of cardioprotective diet in patients with recent acute myocardial infarction: results of one year follow up. *BMJ, 304*, 1015–1019.
4. de Lorgeril, M., Renaud, S., Mamelle, N., Salen, P., Martin, J. L., & Monjaud, I. *et al.* (1994). Mediterranean alpha-linolenic acid-rich diet in secondary prevention of coronary heart disease. *Lancet, 343*, 1454–1459.
5. Faergeman, O., & Grundy, S. M. (2001). *Cholesterol, lipoproteins and coronary heart disease. Dyslipidemia as a health problem: Oxford Textbook of Endocrinology*. Oxford, New York, Toronto: Oxford University Press.
6. Wood, D., De Backer, G., Faergeman, O., Graham, I., Mancia, G., & Pyörälä, K. (1998). Prevention of coronary heart disease in clinical practice: Recommendations of the Second Joint Task Force of European and other societies on coronary prevention. *European Heart Journal, 19*, 1453–1503.
7. Williams, C., McColl, K., & Cowburn, G. (2002). *Food, Nutrition and Cardiovascular Disease Prevention in the European Region: Challenges for the New Millenium. European Heart Network's Nutrition Expert Group* (Ed.). Brussels, European Heart Network.

8. National Cholesterol Education Program Expert Panel (2001). Third Report of the Expert Panel on Detection, Evaluation, and Treatment of High Blood Cholesterol in Adults (Adult Treatment Panel III) Full Report. World Wide Web. 17-5-2002.

9. Nestle, M. (2002). *Food politics. How the food industry influences nutrition and health.* Berkeley: University of California Press.

10. Janus, E. D., Postiglione, A., Singh, R. B., & Lewis, B. (1996). The modernization of Asia. Implications for coronary heart disease. Council on Arteriosclerosis of the International Society and Federation of Cardiology. *Circulation, 94* (11), 2671–2673.

11. Brunet, M., Guy, F., Pilbeam, D., Mackaye, H. T., Likius, A., & Ahounta, D. *et al.* (2002). A new hominid from the Upper Miocene of Chad, Central Africa. *Nature, 418* (6894), 145–151.

12. Diamond, J. (1997). *Guns, germs, and steel: The fates of human societies.* New York, London: W. W. Norton & Company.

13. Cordain, L., Eaton, S. B., Miller, J. B., Mann, N., & Hill, K. (2002). The paradoxical nature of hunter-gatherer diets: meat-based, yet non-atherogenic. *Eur. J. Clin. Nutr., 56* (Suppl. 1), S42-S52.

14. Nestle, M. (1999). Animal versus plant foods in human diets and health: Is the historical record unequivocal? *Proc. Nutr. Soc., 58* (2), 211–218.

15. Drewnowski, A. (1997). Taste preferences and food intake. *Annu. Rev. Nutr., 17,* 237–253.

16. Birch, L. L. (1999). Development of food preferences. *Annu. Rev. Nutr., 19,* 41–62.

17. Rozin, P. (2000). The psychology of food and food choice. In: K. F. Kiple, & K. C. Ornelas (Eds), *The Cambridge world of food* (pp. 1476–1486). Cambridge: Cambridge University Press.

18. Kiple, K. F. (1996). The history of disease. In: R. Porter (Ed.), *The Cambridge illustrated history of medicine* (pp. 16–51). Cambridge: Cambridge University Press.

19. Porter, R. (1997). *The greatest benefit to mankind: A medical history of humanity from antiquity to the present* (paperback 1999 ed.). London: HarperCollins.

20. Zimmer, C. (2001). Genetic trees reveal disease origins. *Science, 292,* 1090–1093.

21. Labarthe, D. R. (1998). *Epidemiology and prevention of cardiovascular diseases: A global challenge.* Gaithersburg, Maryland: Aspen Publishers, Inc.

22. Darwin C. (1998). *The origin of species by means of natural selection or the preservation of favored races in the struggle for life* (Modern Library Paperback ed.). New York: The Modern Library.

23. Doolittle, W. F. (2000). Uprooting the tree of life. *Scientific American, 282,* 90–95.

24. Lewontin, R. (2000). *The triple helix: Gene, organism, and environment.* Cambridge, Massachusetts and London, England: Harvard University Press.

25. Simoons, F. J. (1970). Primary adult lactose intolerance and the milking habit: A problem in biologic and cultural interrelations. II. A culture historical hypothesis. *Am. J. Dig. Dis., 15,* 695–710.

26. Patterson, K. D. (2000). Lactose intolerance. In: K. F. Kiple, & K. C. Ornelas (Eds). *The Cambridge world history of food* (pp. 1057–1062). Cambridge: Cambridge University Press.

27. Weinberg, R. O. (1999). Apolipoprotein A-IV-2 allele: association of its worldwide distribution with adult persistence of lactase and speculation on its function and origin. *Genetic Epidemiology, 17*, 285–297.

28. Newcomer, A. D. (2000). Milk, lactase, and gene distribution. *Digestive Diseases, 23*, 961–962.

29. Johnson, J. D., Simoons, F. J., Hurwitz, R., Grange, A., Sinatra, F. R., & Sunshine, P. *et al.* (1978). Lactose malabsorption among adult Indians of the Great Basin and American Southwest. *Am. J. Clin. Nutr., 31*, 381–387.

30. World Agriculture: Towards 2010 (1995). *An FAO study*. Chichester: John Wiley & Sons.

31. During, M. J., Xu, R., Young, D., Kaplitt, M. G., Sherwin, R. S., & Leone, P. (1998). Peroral gene therapy of lactose intolerance using an adeno-associated virus vector. *Nature Medicine, 4*, 1131–1135.

32. Faergeman, O. (2000). Lactase persistence, milk consumption and coronary artery disease. *Atherosclerosis, 150* (Suppl. 1), S8.

33. Neel, J. V. (1999). The "thrifty genotype" in 1998. *Nutrition Reviews, 57*, S2–S9.

Chapter 6

1. Waltner-Toews, D., & Lang, T. (2000). A new conceptual base for food and agricultural policy: the emerging model of links between agriculture, food, health, and environment and society. *Global Change and Human Health, 1* (2), 116–130.

2. Williams, C., McColl, K., & Cowburn, G. (2002). *Food, Nutrition and Cardiovascular Disease Prevention in the European Region: Challenges for the New Millenium*. European Heart Network's Nutrition Expert Group (Ed.). Brussels, European Heart Network.

3. Kjærgaard, T. (1994). *The Danish revolution, 1500–1800: An ecohistorical interpretation*. Cambridge, New York, Melbourne: Cambridge University Press.

4. Davies, N. (1996). *Europe: A history*. Oxford, New York: Oxford University Press.

5. McKay, J. P., Hill, B. D., & Buckler, J. (1999). The Revolution in Energy and Industry. In: A. Shaw, D. Anderson, L. Rothrauff, & C. M. Horn (Eds). *A history of western society* (Vol. C). *From the revolutionary era to the present* (pp. 724–753). Boston, New York: Houghton Mifflin Company.

6. Wright A. (2000). Personal communication.

7. Courtois, S., Werth, N., Panné, J-L., Paczkowski, A., Bartosek, K., & Margolin, J-L. (1999). *The black book of communism: Crimes, terror, repression*. Cambridge, Massachusetts; London: Harvard University Press.

8. Traktat om Oprettelse af Det Europæiske Økonomiske Fælleskab (1972). Copenhagen: Markedssekretariatet, Udenrigsministeriet.

9. Nestle, M. (2002). *Food politics. How the food industry influences nutrition and health*. Berkeley: University of California Press.

10. Regeringens forebyggelsesprogram (1989). *Programdel*. Copenhagen: Sundheds-ministeriet.

11. Handbook of Energy Utilization in Agriculture (1980). Boca Raton, Florida: CRC Press.

12. Lappé, F. M. (1971). *Diet for a small planet*. New York: Ballantine Books, Inc.

13. Jackson, W. (1985). *New roots for agriculture* (2nd ed.). Lincoln: University of Nebraska Press.

14. Darwin, C. (1998). The origin of species by means of natural selection or the preservation of favored races in the struggle for life (Modern Library Paperback ed.). New York: The Modern Library.

15. Robinson, R. A. (1996). *Return to resistance: Breeding crops to reduce pesticide dependence*. Davis, California: agAccess.

16. Andrews, N. J., Farrington, C. P., Cousens, S. N., Smith, P. G., Ward, H., & Knight, R. S. *et al.* (2000). Incidence of variant Creutzfeldt-Jakob disease in the U.K. *Lancet, 356* (9228), 481–482.

17. Porter, R. (1997). *The greatest benefit to mankind. A medical history of humanity from antiquity to the present* (Paperback 1999 ed.). London: Harper-Collins.

18. World Agriculture: Towards 2010 (1995). *An FAO study*. Chichester: John Wiley & Sons.

19. Pinstrup-Andersen, P., Pandya-Loch, R., & Rosegrant, M. W. (1999). *World food prospects: Critical issues for the early twenty-first century*. Washington D.C., International Food Policy Research Institute.

20. The Global Burden of Disease (1996). Cambridge: Harvard University Press.

21. Cordain, L. (1999). Cereal grains: Humanity's double-edged sword. In: A. P. Simopoulos (Ed.), *Evolutionary aspects of nutrition and health. diet, exercise, genetics and chronic disease* (pp. 19–73). Basel: Karger.

22. Russel, J. B., & Rychlik, J. L. (2001). Factors that alter rumen microbial ecology. *Science, 292*, 1119–1122.

23. Nissinen, A., Berrios, X., & Puska, P. (2001). Community-based noncommunicable disease interventions: lessons from developed countries for developing ones. *Bull. World Health Organ., 79* (10), 963–970.

24. Pekka, P., Pirjo, P., & Ulla, U. (2002). Influencing public nutrition for non-communicable disease prevention: from community intervention to national programme — experiences from Finland. *Public Health Nutr., 5* (1A), 245–251.

25. Bettcher, D. W., Puska, P., & Yach, D. (2002). Personal communication.

26. Agricultural Policies in OECD Countries (2002). Monitoring and evaluation 2002. Highlights: Full report has ISBN 9264191992. Organisation for Economic Co-operation and Development.

27. Forsdahl A. (1977). Are poor living conditions in childhood and adolescence an important risk factor for arteriosclerotic heart disease? *British Journal of Preventive and Social Medicine, 31*, 91–95.

28. Forsen, T., Eriksson, J. G., Tuomilehto, J., Osmund, C., & Barker, D. J. (1999). Growth in utero and during childhood among women who develop coronary heart disease: Longitudinal study. *BMJ, 319*, 1403–1407.

29. The Bichel-Committee (1999). Report from the Main Committee to Assess the Overall Consequences of Phasing out the Use of Pesticides. Copenhagen, Danish Environmental Protection Agency (Ministry of Environment and Energy).
30. Special Report No 8/2000 on the Community measures for the disposal of butterfat accompanied by the Commission's replies. Official Journal of the European Communities C 132[43]. 12-5-2000.
31. Greider W. (2000). *The last farm crisis: The nation.*
32. The curse of factory farms (2002). *International Herald Tribune*, (Aug. 31), 6.
33. Dørge H. (2001). Det hvide guld. *Weekendavisen Berlingske*, (Sep. 28), 1–5.
34. Hundsbæk, T., Hoffmann, T., & Schilling, B. (2001). Steff-Houlberg giver op. *Politiken*, (Nov 3), 10.
34. Mørch, T. Y., & Hundsbæk, T. (2002). Opgør om leverpostej-patent. *Politiken*, (May 9).

Chapter 7

1. Koch, L. (2000). *Tvangssterilisation i Danmark 1929–1967.* København: Gyldendal.
2. Goldstein, J. L., & Brown, M. S. (1979). The LDL receptor locus and the genetics of familial hypercholesterolemia. *Annu. Rev. Genet.*, *13*, 259–289.
3. Innerarity, T. L., Weisgraber, K. H., Arnold, K. S., Mahley, R. W., Krauss, R. M., & Vega, G. L. *et al.* (1987). Familial defective apolipoprotein B-100: Low density lipoproteins with abnormal receptor binding. *Proc. Natl. Acad. Sci. USA*, *84*, 6919–6923.
4. Garcia, C. K., Wilund, K., Arca, M., Zuliani, G., Fellin, R., Maioli, M. *et al.* (2001). Autosomal recessive hypercholesterolemia caused by mutations in a putative LDL receptor adaptor protein. *Science*, *292* (5520), 1394–1398.
5. Jensen, H. K., Jensen, L. G., Meinertz, H., Hansen, P. S., Gregersen, N., & Faergeman, O. (1999). Spectrum of LDL receptor gene mutations in Denmark: Implications for molecular diagnostic strategy in heterozygous familial hypercholesterolemia. *Atherosclerosis*, *146* (2), 337–344.
6. Jensen, H. K., Jensen, T. G., Faergeman, O., Jensen, L. G., Andresen, B. S., & Corydon, M. J. *et al.* (1997). Two mutations in the same low-density lipoprotein receptor allele act in synergy to reduce receptor function in heterozygous familial hypercholesterolemia. *Hum. Mutat.*, *9* (5), 437–444.
7. Andersen, L. K., Jensen, H. K., Juul, S., & Faergeman, O. (1997). Patients' attitudes toward detection of heterozygous familial hypercholesterolemia. *Arch. Intern. Med.*, *157* (5), 553–560.
8. Scandinavian Simvastatin Survival Study Group (1994). Randomised trial of cholesterol lowering in 4444 patients with coronary heart disease: The Scandinavian Simvastatin Survival Study (4S). *Lancet*, *344* (8934), 1383–1389.
9. Utermann, G. (1975). Isolation and partial characterization of an arginine-rich apolipoprotein from human plasma very-low-density lipoproteins: Apolipoprotein E. *Hoppe Seylers Z. Physiol. Chem.*, *356* (7), 1113–1121.

10. Mahley, R. W., & Rall, S. C. Jr. (2000). Apolipoprotein E: Far more than a lipid transport protein. *Annual Review of Genomics and Human Genetics*, *1*, 507–537.

11. Berg, K. (1963). A new serum type system in man — the Lp system. *Acta Pathol. Microbiol. Scand.*, *59*, 369–382.

12. Gaw, A., & Hobbs, H. H. (1999). Lipoprotein(a). In: D. J. Betteridge, D. R. Illingworth, & J. Shepherd (Eds), *Lipoproteins in health and disease.* (pp. 87–109). London, Sydney, Auckland: Arnold.

13. Hobbs, H. H., & White, A. L. (1999). Lipoprotein(a): Intrigues and insights. *Curr. Opin. Lipidol.*, *10* (3), 225–236.

14. Gerdes, L. U., Gerdes, C., Kervinen, K., Savolainen, M., Klausen, I. C., & Hansen, P. S. *et al.* (2000). The apolipoprotein ε4 allele determines prognosis and the effect on prognosis of simvastatin in survivors of myocardial infarction: A substudy of the Scandinavian Simvastatin Survival Study. *Circulation*, *101*, 1366–1371.

15. Schwartz M., Lund, E. G., & Russel, D. W. (1998). Two 7α-hydroxylase enzymes in bile acid synthesis. *Current Opinion in Lipidology*, *9*, 113–118.

16. Tautz, D. (2000). A genetic uncertainty problem. *TIG*, *16*, 475–477.

17. Strohman, R. C. (1993). Ancient genomes, wise bodies, unhealthy people: limits of a genetic paradigm in biology and medicine. *Persp. Biol. Med.*, *37*, 112–145.

18. The Global Burden of Disease (1996). Cambridge: Harvard University Press.

19. Templeton, A. R. (1999). Use of evolutionary theory in the Human Genome Project. *Ann. Rev. Ecol. Syst.*, *30*, 23–49.

20. Templeton, A. R., Clark, A. G., Weiss, K. M., Nickerson, D. A., Boerwinkle, E., & Sing, C. F. (2000). Recombinational and mutational hotspots within the human lipoprotein lipase gene. *American Journal of Human Genetics*, *66*, 69–83.

21. Gene-mappers take new aim at diseases. *The New York Times*, (30-10-2002). Internet Communication.

22. Weiss, K. M., & Clark, A. G. (2002). Linkage disequilibrium and the mapping of complex human traits. *Trends Genet.*, *18* (1), 19–24.

23. Gretarsdottir, S., Sveinbjornsdottir, S., Jonsson, H. H., Jakobsson, F., Einarsdottir, E., & Agnarsson, U. *et al.* (2002). Localization of a susceptibility gene for common forms of stroke to 5q12. *Am. J. Hum. Genet.*, *70* (3), 593–603.

24. Stengård, J. H., Clark, A. G., Weiss, K. M., Kardia, S., Nickerson, D. A., & Salomaa, V. *et al.* (2002). Contributions of 18 additional DNA sequence variations in the gene encoding apolipoprotein E to explaining variation in quantitative measures of lipid metabolism. *Am. J. Hum. Genet.*, *71* (3), 501–517.

25. Abbott A. (1999). Alliance of U.S. labs plans to build map of cell signalling pathways. *Nature*, *402*, 219–220.

26. Smaglik, P. (2000). For my next trick . . . *Nature*, *407*, 828–829.

27. Coveney, P., & Highfield, R. (1995). *Frontiers of complexity: The search for order in a chaotic world*. New York: Fawcett Columbine.

28. Sing, C. F., Zerba, K. E., & Reilly, S. L. Traversing the biological complexity in the hierarchy between genome and CAD endpoints in the population at large. *Clinical Genetics*, *46*, 6–14.

29. Lewontin, R. (2000). The triple helix. gene, organism, and environment. Cambridge, Massachusetts and London, England: Harvard University Press.
30. Strohman, R. (2000). Upcoming Revolution in Biology. In: C. Walker (Ed.), *Made not born: The troubling world of biotechnology* (pp. 108–118). San Francisco: Sierra Club Books.
31. Kjærgaard, T. (1991). *Den danske revolution 1500–1800: En økohistorisk tolkning.* København: Gyldendal.
32. Daws, G., & Fujita, M. (1999). *Archipelago: The islands of Indonesia. From the nineteenth-century discoveries of Alfred Russel Wallace to the fate of the forests and reefs in the twenty-first century.* Berkeley, Los Angeles, London: University of California Press.
33. Darwin, C. (1998). *The origin of species by means of natural selection or the preservation of favored races in the struggle for Life* (Modern Library Paperback ed.). New York: The Modern Library, 1998.
34. Gould, S. J. (2002). *The structure of evolutionary theory.* Cambridge, Massachusetts: Belknap Press of Harvard University Press.
35. Dawkins, R. (1986). *The blind watchmaker.* London: Penguin Books.
36. Goodwin, B. (2001). *How the leopard changed its spots: The evolution of complexity. Princeton: Princeton University Press.*
37. Greenspan, R. J. (2001). The flexible genome. *Nat. Rev. Genet., 2* (5), 383–387.

Chapter 8

1. Frank, L. (2000). Englene over Øresund. *Weekendavisen Berlingske*, (Feb. 18), 6.
2. Frank, L. (2002). Biotechnology in the Medicon Valley. *Nat. Biotechnol., 20* (5), 433–435.
3. Werth, B. (1994). *The billion dollar molecule: One company's quest for the perfect drug.* New York, London, Toronto, Sydney, Tokyo, Singapore: Simon & Schuster.
4. Borger J. (2002). "Clean-up" swept under the carpet. *The Guardian Weekly*, (Nov. 7), 6.
5. Essick, K. (2002). Start-ups struggled in 2001. *The Wall Street Journal*, (Jan. 4), 9–14.
6. Press, E., & Washburn, J. (2000). The Kept University. *The Atlantic Monthly, 285* (3), 39–54.
7. Arbejdsgruppen vedrørende samfinansierede forskningsprojekter (2000). *Samarbejdsaftaler mellem universitetet og erhvervsvirksomheder.* Copenhagen: Forskningsministeriet.
8. Vogel, G. (2002). Germany's elite tie knot with big pharma. *Science*, (295), 950–951.
9. Nelsen, L. (1998). The rise of intellectual property protection in the American university. *Science Magazine, 279*, 1460–1461.
10. Frank, L. (2000). Støtte til eliten. *Weekendavisen Berlingske*, 1–7.
11. Comroe, J. H. Jr. (1971). Contributions of basic research to clinical medicine. *Chest, 59*, 208–211.

12. Berry, W. (2000). *Life is a miracle. An essay against modern superstition.* Washington, D.C.: Cunterpoint.
13. Seidelin, M., & Ilsøe, T. M. (2001). Nyt styre til universiteterne. *Politiken*, (Dec. 27; Sect. Indland), 4.
14. Charles, D. (2001). *Lords of the harvest: Biotech, big money, and the future of food.* Cambridge, Massachusetts: Perseus Publishing.
15. Pimentel, D., & Raven, P. H. (2001). Bt corn pollen impacts on nontarget Lepidoptera: Assessment of effects in nature. *PNAS, 97*, 8198–8199.
16. Pinstrup-Andersen, P., Pandya-Loch, R., & Rosegrant, M. W. (1999). *World food prospects: Critical issues for the early twenty-first century.* Washington, D.C.: International Food Policy Research Institute.
17. James, C. (2001). *Global review of commercialized transgenic crops: 2000. ISAAA briefs no. 23 — 2001.* Ithaca, NY: International Service for the Acquisition of Agri-biotech Applications.
18. Ehrenfeld, D. (1993). *Beginning again: People and nature in the new millenium.* New York, Oxford: Oxford University Press.

Chapter 9

1. Porter, R. (1997). *The greatest benefit to mankind: A medical history of humanity from antiquity to the present* (Paperback 1999 ed.). London: HarperCollins.
2. Fukuyama, F. (2002). *Our posthuman future: Consequences of the biotechnology revolution.* New York: Farra, Straus and Giroux.
3. Hall, S. S. (2002). Human cloning: President's bioethics council delivers. *Science, 297* (5580), 322–324.
4. Sackett, D. L., Richardson, W. S., Rosenberg, W., & Haynes, R. B. (1997). *Evidence-based medicine. How to practice and teach EBM.* New York: Churchill-Livingstone.
5. Hulley, S., Grady, D., Bush, T., Furberg, C., Herrington, D., & Riggs, B. *et al.* (1998). Randomized trial of estrogen plus progestin for secondary prevention of coronary heart disease in postmenopausal women: Heart and Estrogen/progestin Replacement Study (HERS) Research Group. *JAMA, 280* (7), 605–613.
6. Grady, D., Herrington, D., Bittner, V., Blumenthal, R., Davidson, M., & Hlatky, M. *et al.* (2002). Cardiovascular disease outcomes during 6.8 years of hormone therapy: Heart and Estrogen/progestin Replacement Study follow-up (HERS II). *JAMA, 288* (1), 49–57.
7. (2002). Risks and benefits of estrogen plus progestin in healthy postmenopausal women: Principal results from the Women's Health Initiative randomized controlled trial. *JAMA, 288* (3), 321–333.
8. The Cardiac Arrhythmia Suppression Trial (CAST) Investigators (1989). Preliminary report: effect of encainide and flecainide on mortality in a randomized trial of arrhythmia suppression after myocardial infarction. *New England Journal of Medicine, 321*, 406–412.

9. Heart Protection Study Collaborative Group (2002). MRC/BHF Heart Protection Study: Randomised placebo-controlled trial of cholesterol lowering with simvastatin in 20,536 high-risk individuals: a randomised placebo-controlled trial. *Lancet*, *360*, 7–22.
10. Evidence Based Cardiology (1998). BMJ Publishing Group.
11. Inglesby, T. V., Henderson, D. A., Bartlett, J. G., Ascher, M. S., Eitzen, E., & Friedlander, A. M. *et al.* (1999). Anthrax as a biological weapon. Medical and public health management. *JAMA*, *281*, 1735–1745.
12. Evans, R. G. (1997). Sharing the burden, containing the cost: Fundamental conflicts in health care finance. In: T. J. Litman, & L. S. Robins (Eds), *Health Politics and Policy* (3rd ed.) (pp. 265–287). Albany: Delmar Publishers Inc.
13. U.K. Prospective Diabetes Study (UKPDS) (1998). Intensive blood-glucose control with sulphonylureas or insulin compared to conventional treatment and risk of complications in patients with type 2 diabetes. *Lancet*, *352*, 837–853.
14. Wessely, S., Rose, S., & Bisson, J. (2000). Brief psychological interventions ("debriefing)" for trauma-related symptoms and the prevention of post traumatic stress disorder. *Cochrane Database Syst. Rev.*, (2), CD000560.
15. Kenardy, J. (2000). The current status of psychological debriefing. *BMJ*, *321*, 1032–1033.
16. Færgeman, O. (2002). Evidensbaseret medicin, sundhedspolitik og administrativ kontrol med lægers arbejde. *Ugeskift for Læger*, *164*, 1538–1543.

Chapter 10

1. Evans, R. G. (1997). Sharing the burden, containing the cost: Fundamental conflicts in health care finance. In: T. J. Litman, L. S. Robins (Eds), *Health Politics and Policy* (3rd ed.) (pp. 265–287). Albany: Delmar Publishers Inc.
2. Mainz, J. (1996). *Problemidentifikation og Kvalitetsvurdering i Sundhedsvæsenet.* København: Munksgaard.
3. Faergeman, O. (1998). Guidelines for the prevention of coronary artery disease: Relating local needs to local initiatives. *Dis Mange Health Outcomes*, *4*, 217–224.
4. Goodwin, J. S. (1999). Geriatrics and the limits of modern medicine. *New England Journal of Medicine*, *340*, 1283–1285.
5. Flyvbjerg, B. (1991). *Rationalitet og Magt.* Odense, Denmark: Akademisk Forlag.
6. Topol, E. J., & Califf, R. M. (1998). Quality of care in cardiovascular medicine. In: E. J. Topol (Ed.), *Textbook of cardiovascular medicine* (pp. 1119–1134). Philadelphia, New York: Lippincott-Raven.
7. Lauer, M. S., & Fortinm D. F. (1998). Databases in cardiology. In: E. J. Topol (Ed.), *Textbook of Cardiovascular Medicine* (pp. 1083–1106). Philadelphia, New York: Lippincott-Raven.
8. Issel, L. M., & Kahn, D. (1998). The economic value of caring. *Health Care Mangement Review*, *23* (4), 43–53.
9. Wynia, M. K., Cummins, D. S., VanGeest, J. B., & Wilson, I. B. (2000). Physician manipulation of reimbursement rules for patients: between a rock and a hard place. *JAMA*, *283* (14), 1858–1865.

10. (1988). Randomised trial of intravenous streptokinase, oral aspirin, both, or neither among 17,187 cases of suspected acute myocardial infarction: ISIS-2. ISIS-2 (Second International Study of Infarct Survival) Collaborative Group. *Lancet, 2* (8607), 349–360.

Conclusions

1. Leibowitz, J. O. (1970). *The history of coronary heart disease*. London, Wellcome Institute of the History of Medicine.
2. The World Health Report 2002 (2002). *Reducing risks, promoting healthy life*. Geneva: World Health Organization.
3. Williams, C., McColl, K., & Cowburn, G. (2002). *Food, nutrition and cardiovascular disease prevention in the european region: Challenges for the new millenium.* European Heart Network's Nutrition Expert Group (Ed). Brussels: European Heart Network.

Appendix 1: A Crash Course in Coronary Artery Disease

Arteries are tubes that channel oxygenated blood from the lungs and heart to the various organs of the body. The main artery is called the aorta. It channels blood into a whole tree of progressively finer arteries. The first two arteries branching off from the aorta are the coronary arteries, which surround the heart like a corona, or crown, before they send smaller branches into the heart muscle to supply it with oxygen and nutrients. Atherosclerosis is a disease that thickens and narrows certain arteries including the coronary arteries. Atherosclerosis is a composite word. *Athere* is the Greek word for porridge, and *skleros* is the Greek word for hard. If you examine the artery that caused someone to suffer from some kind of atherosclerotic disease, you will find certain parts of the artery in which a little pocket of porridge has been formed in the wall of the artery. The porridge has the consistency of toothpaste. Usually it is not in contact with the blood flowing through the artery, because it is encapsulated in hard tissue. If the hard tissue weakens, however, it can rupture so that the porridge oozes into the blood. When that happens, blood forms a clot or a thrombus. Sometimes the clot just further narrows the artery, but at other times it closes the artery off completely. Whereas atherosclerosis forms gradually, in a matter of months and years, clotting is rapid. It occurs in a matter of minutes and hours.

Atherosclerosis can narrow the aorta and some of the larger branches of the aorta. If it narrows or closes off the arteries to the brain, it causes a stroke. If it narrows an artery to the legs, it causes muscle pain when walking, and if it closes the artery off completely it causes gangrene of the leg. If it closes off an artery to the intestine, it causes gangrene of part of the intestine. And if it narrows or closes off an artery to the heart, it causes chest pain or gangrene of part of the heart muscle. The chest pain is called angina pectoris, and gangrene of the heart muscle is called a myocardial infarct. Myocardium means heart muscle, and an infarct is the dead part of a muscle or any other organ deprived of its supply of blood. If the patient survives an infarct in the heart, the dead part of the heart muscle is replaced by scar tissue.

The heart is a hollow muscle that pumps blood. The right side of the heart pumps blood through the lungs, where it gives off carbon dioxide and picks up oxygen. The left side of the heart then pumps the blood through the rest of the body, where it gives off oxygen and picks up carbon dioxide. Blood also transports nutrients, waste products, salts and hormones between organs. Arteries channel blood away from the heart, and after it has passed through the tiniest of tubes called capillaries, the blood is again channeled back to the heart through the veins.

Patients with atherosclerosis in one part of the arterial tree virtually always have atherosclerosis elsewhere in the tree. Most patients who have survived a stroke due to atherosclerosis of one of the arteries to the brain will later die of atherosclerosis of the coronary arteries. Similarly, most patients with pain in the legs due to atherosclerosis of one of the arteries to the legs will also later die of a myocardial infarct due to atherosclerosis of the coronary arteries. That is the reason why deaths due to myocardial infarcts are a rough measure of how much atherosclerosis there is in various populations across the planet.

Appendix 2: A Mini-course on Fats

Fats are esters of glycerol and fatty acids or related organic compounds. Fatty acids can vary substantially in length, and they are said to be "saturated", if they contain as many hydrogen atoms as possible. They are, in effect, saturated with hydrogen. Fatty acids lacking two or more hydrogen atoms are unsaturated. If only two adjacent carbon atoms each lack a hydrogen atom, the fatty acids is monounsaturated. If several pairs of adjacent carbon atoms lack hydrogen atoms, the fatty acid is polyunsaturated. By convention, the unsaturated bond between the carbon atoms is indicated by an equal sign (=). Below are some examples.

A saturated fatty acid (palmitic):

CH3-CH2-CH2-CH2-CH2-CH2-CH2-CH2-CH2-CH2-CH2-CH2-CH2-CH2-CH2-COOH

A monounsaturated fatty acid (oleic):

CH3-CH2-CH2-CH2-CH2-CH2-CH2-CH2-CH = CH-CH2-CH2-CH2-CH2-CH2-CH2-CH2-COOH

A polyunsaturated fatty acid (α-linolenic):

CH3-CH2-CH = CH-CH2-CH2-CH2-CH2-CH = CH-CH2-CH = CH-CH2-CH2-CH2-CH2-COOH

The first and only unsaturated bond in oleic acid is between carbon atoms 9 and 10 (counted from the methyl group), whereas the first unsaturated bond in α-linolenic acid is between carbon atoms 3 and 4. Oleic acid is therefore also called an *n*-9 monounsaturated fatty acid, whereas α-linolenic acid is called an n-3 polyunsaturated fatty acid.

Glycerol   CH2OH
                                            CHOH
                                            CH2OH

A molecule of triglyceride is produced when 3 fatty acids bond to glycerol. Each fatty acid forms an ester bond between its carboxyl group (–COOH) and one of the hydroxyl groups (–OH) groups of glycerol. Triglyceride is one of many kinds of fat. If the fatty acids are mainly unsaturated, triglyceride is fluid at room temperature, an oil. If the fatty acids are mainly saturated, the fat is relatively solid at room temperature. Butter is an example of hard fat.

The culprits that cause atherosclerosis are the long saturated fatty acids, such as palmitic acid, and a kind of unsaturated fatty acids called trans-unsaturated fatty acids ("trans-fats"). The spatial arrangement of an unsaturated bond, and of the whole molecule, of trans-unsaturated fatty acids has been changed from its natural form.

Subject Index